REMOTE CARDIOLOGY CONSULTATIONS USING ADVANCED MEDICAL TECHNOLOGY

NATO Science Series

A series presenting the results of scientific meetings supported under the NATO Science Programme.

The series is published by IOS Press and Springer Science and Business Media in conjunction with the NATO Public Diplomacy Division.

Sub-Series

I. Life and Behavioural Sciences	IOS Press
II. Mathematics, Physics and Chemistry	Springer Science and Business Media
III. Computer and Systems Sciences	IOS Press
IV. Earth and Environmental Sciences	Springer Science and Business Media
V. Science and Technology Policy	IOS Press

The NATO Science Series continues the series of books published formerly as the NATO ASI Series.

The NATO Science Programme offers support for collaboration in civil science between scientists of countries of the Euro-Atlantic Partnership Council. The types of scientific meeting generally supported are "Advanced Study Institutes" and "Advanced Research Workshops", although other types of meeting are supported from time to time. The NATO Science Series collects together the results of these meetings. The meetings are co-organized by scientists from NATO countries and scientists from NATO's Partner countries – countries of the CIS and Central and Eastern Europe.

Advanced Study Institutes are high-level tutorial courses offering in-depth study of the latest advances in a field.
Advanced Research Workshops are expert meetings aimed at critical assessment of a field, and identification of directions for future action.

As a consequence of the restructuring of the NATO Science Programme in 1999, the NATO Science Series has been re-organized and there are currently five sub-series as noted above. Please consult the following web sites for information on previous volumes published in the series, as well as details of earlier sub-series:

http://www.nato.int/science
http://www.springeronline.nl
http://www.iospress.nl
http://www.wtv-books.de/nato_pco.htm

Series I. Life and Behavioural Sciences – Vol. 372   ISSN: 1566-7693

Remote Cardiology Consultations Using Advanced Medical Technology

Applications for NATO Operations

Edited by

Ivica Klapan

*Zagreb University School of Medicine & Clinical Hospital Center Zagreb,
Zagreb, Croatia*

and

Ronald Poropatich

*Telemedicine and Advanced Technology Research Center, United States Army
Medical Research and Materiel Command, Fort Detrick, MD, USA*

/OS
Press

Amsterdam • Berlin • Oxford • Tokyo • Washington, DC

Published in cooperation with NATO Public Diplomacy Division

Proceedings of the NATO Advanced Research Workshop on Remote Cardiology Consultations
Using Advanced Medical Technology – Applications for NATO Operations
Zagreb, Croatia
13–16 September 2005

ISBN 1-58603-657-2
Library of Congress Control Number: 2006935042

Publisher
IOS Press
Nieuwe Hemweg 6B
1013 BG Amsterdam
Netherlands
fax: +31 20 687 0019
e-mail: order@iospress.nl

Distributor in the UK and Ireland
Gazelle Books Services Ltd.
White Cross Mills
Hightown
Lancaster LA1 4XS
United Kingdom
fax: +44 1524 63232
e-mail: sales@gazellebooks.co.uk

Distributor in the USA and Canada
IOS Press, Inc.
4502 Rachael Manor Drive
Fairfax, VA 22032
USA
fax: +1 703 323 3668
e-mail: iosbooks@iospress.com

IOS Press, 2006

Preface

The Role of Advanced Medical Technology in Cardiology

NATO operations have expanded in recent years, and the old Cold War concept of "every nation provides its own medical support" is no longer tenable, nor is it NATO policy. In the future, NATO medical care will often be provided on a multinational basis, especially in case of emergencies such as NATO response to natural or man-made disasters or to terrorist actions. Even though deployed military personnel are usually young and relatively healthy, this is not the case for all those who may be provided care by NATO medical personnel. The pressures to "shorten the logistics tail", coupled with the shortage of trained cardiologists in most of our nations, has and will continue to preclude the routine deployment of Cardiologists to all NATO operational missions. However, the need to provide services during these missions remains very real. Even following a natural disaster or exposure to toxic agents, the ability to distinguish a cardiac event from other causes of chest pain can be life-saving, and appropriate diagnosis will lead to improved survival, reduced inappropriate use of medical capabilities, and decreased inappropriate evacuation of patients.

Acute coronary syndromes (e.g. angina and myocardial infarction) and associated cardiac emergency conditions (e.g. arrthymias) remain the leading cause of death among industrialized nations, and deployed military personnel are certainly not immune from this threat. New diagnostic (e.g. portable ultrasound) and treatment modalities (e.g. fibrinolytic agents) have greatly improved the survival of the cardiac diseased patient, assuming the diagnosis can be made rapidly. Associated improvements in advanced medical technology and tele-communications, have enabled cardiac patients in remote or austere environments access to specialty consultation, even though the Cardiologist may be located elsewhere. This capability has resulted in decreased morbidity and mortality. Examples of this kind of second opinion consultation occur in the field of telehealth or telemedicine. In this case, cardiac patients in a remote site can undergo testing and evaluation with an electrocardiogram (ECG) or echocardiogram (ECHO) captured in a digital format, which can then be forwarded over commercial communication networks to a medical center for interpretation by a cardiac specialist. Supplementation of this capability with real time transmission of a patient examination with heart sounds (tele-stethoscopy) or videoteleconferencing (VTC), may augment the medical evaluation and provide the remote medical provider immediate referral recommendations that can be life-saving.

In the military setting, deployed NATO forces in remote locations (e.g. Kosovo) are comprised of young as well as middle-aged forces that are susceptible to suffering an acute cardiac event. These deployed sites typically do not have a cardiologist available at the remote medical treatment facility. Often, if two-way voice communication is established, cardiac specialists can be consulted with a limited view of the cardiac patient. Increased bandwidth availability is now becoming possible in remote deployed environments and permitting the use of tele-consultation in a variety of medical disciplines. Advanced medical technologies (digital cardiac ECG and ECHO machines) in the field of cardiology have been developed and are routine in the management of cardiac patients. Other enabling technologies include advances in compression of digital data allowing transmission of large data files over low bandwidth systems (e.g. Internet) as well as increased availability of large bandwidth systems using satellite technologies.

Many nations and agencies currently have ongoing research in this field, including the US, France, Spain, the Netherlands, Norway, Croatia, the European Commission, and the World Bank. There is a scientific need to bring many of these researchers together to discuss mechanisms for interoperability, and to begin the discussions about Telecardiology Standardization to allow regional and other multinational mutual support. In Croatia, the need for remote tele-cardiology consultation is necessary in order to meet the growing demand for expert medical advice for tourists vacationing in remote islands in the Adriatic Sea who take ill with a cardiac event. To address this concern in Croatia, a World Bank funded initiative in the field of tele-cardiology was approved and work is already underway to meet this need. The Croatian Ministry of Health is the stakeholder organization shepherding this initiative. Likewise, in the US military, transmission of digital ECG's and ECHO images is occurring in medical treatment facilities in the continental United States but infrequently in operational settings such as Iraq or Afghanistan.

In September 2005, a NATO sponsored Advanced Research Workshop (ARW) titled **"Remote Cardiology Consultations Using Advanced Medical Technology – Applications for NATO Operations"** was conducted in Zagreb, Croatia and provided a forum to discuss the advances in diagnostic medical technologies as they apply to the specialty of cardiology. Experiences gained from NATO forces in both garrison and deployed environments were shared. Lessons Learned from an international community in the field of tele-cardiology were identified with far-reaching impact as new systems are developed and deployed in future NATO missions.

The ARW consisted of several panel presentations over three days drawing from experts in health, clinical research, electrical engineering and law. The main focus of the meeting was to:

a. address the clinical need for tele-cardiology in a remote or austere environment;
b. to assess cost-effective technical solutions with "off the shelf" hardware and non-proprietary software;
c. to articulate the human factors challenges in developing regional cardiac consultation;
d. to identify the legal, regulatory, and security concerns for remote tele-consultation; and
e. to develop a business case analysis for tele-cardiology that will allow self-sustainment of services based on sound economic expectations.

The efforts of this meeting culminated in the development of this book which summarizes the current state of Telecardiology as presented by the member participants totalling nearly 60 individuals and representing over 16 NATO and Partner for Peace nations. We thank the meeting participants and the Organizing Committee for their tireless efforts in successfully conducting the meeting and preparing their manuscripts for inclusion in this book. We especially thank the NATO Advisory Panel on Security-Related Civil Science and Technology and the Assistant Secretary General for Public Diplomacy, for their financial award, without which this meeting could never have occurred.

NATO country co-director

COL Ronald Poropatich, MD
US Army Medical Research & Materiel Command
Telemedicine and Advanced Technology Research Center
Fort Detrick, MD, USA

Partner country co-director

Professor Ivica Klapan, MD, PhD
Croatian Telemedicine Society of the Croatian Medical Association (President)
Telemedicine Committee-Ministry of Health and Social Welfare, Republic of Croatia (President)
Department of ORL-H&N Surgery, Zagreb University School of Medicine & Clinical Hospital Center Zagreb, Šalata 4, HR-10000 Zagreb, Croatia

Workshop Organization

Co-directors

NATO-country co-director

COL Poropatich, Ronald, MD
US Army Medical Research & Materiel Command
Telemedicine and Advanced Technology Research Center
Fort Detrick, MD, USA
001-301-619-7967/301-619-2518
poropatich@tatrc.org

Partner-country co-director

Professor Klapan, Ivica, MD, PhD
Croatian Telemedicine Society of the Croatian Medical Association (President)
Telemedicine Committee-Ministry of Health and Social Welfare, Republic of Croatia
    (President)
Department of ORL-H&N Surgery, Zagreb University School of Medicine &
Clinical Hospital Center Zagreb, Šalata 4, HR-10000 Zagreb, Croatia
00385-1-4920038/1-4920630
telmed@mef.hr
www.mef.hr/MODERNRHINOLOGY

Croatian Co-Presidents

Miličić Davor	Professor; President, Croatian Cardiac Society; Vice-President, Croatian Telemedicine Society of the Croatian Medical Association; Vice-President, Telemedicine Committee of the Ministry of Health and Social Welfare, Republic of Croatia
Kovač Mario	Professor, Faculty of Electrical Engineering and Computing, University of Zagreb; Board Member, Croatian Telemedicine Society of the Croatian Medical Association; Member, Telemedicine Committee of the Ministry of Health and Social Welfare, Republic of Croatia

Organizing Committee

Duvančić Sanja	Ministry of Defence Republic of Croatia
Lam David	Secretary, NATO/COMEDS Telemedicine Panel, Brussels (Belgium) University of Maryland School of Medicine; National Study Center for Trauma and Emergency Medical Systems; U.S. Army Telemedicine and Advanced Technology Research Center (TATRC)
Medved Ivan	Secretary, Telemedicine Committee of the Ministry of Health and Social Welfare, Republic of Croatia
Mittermayer Renato	Deputy Minister, Ministry of Health and Social Welfare, Republic of Croatia
Schwarz Dragan	Deputy Minister, Ministry of Science, Republic of Croatia

Contributors

Surname	Initials	Title	Institute
Hernandez Abadia	A	Captain/MD	Ministry of Defence, Madrid (Spain)+++ ahabadia@inicia.es
Barjaktari	G	Professor/MD	Department of Cardiology, University of Prishtina (Kosovo) +++;
Chernysh	P	Professor/MD	Central Military Hospital, Department of Cardiology (Head) (Uzbekistan) +++; chernysh_pavel@mail.ru
Damjanić	L	MSEE	Ericsson Co., Shanghai (China) +++; lorenco@public3.sta.net.cn; lorenco.damjanic@ericsson.co
Delić	M	Professor/MD	Vice President, Bosnian Society of Cardiology; Deptartment of Cardiology, University of Sarajevo (Bosnia and Herzegovina) +++
Goldner	I	MS, Dipl.iur.	igoldner@pravo.hr
Grabar-Kitarović	K	Professor	Minister of Foreign Affairs and European Integrations, Croatian Government, Zagreb (Croatia) +++; glasnogovornik@mvp.hr
Jordanova	M	Professor/MD	Bulgarian Academy of Sciences, Sofia (Member) (Bulgaria)+++; mjordan@bas.bg
Klapan	I	Professor/MD	Croatian Telemedicine Society-Croatian Medical Association (President); Telemedicine Committee-Ministry of Health and Social Welfare (President); Department of ORL-H&N Surgery, Zagreb University School of Medicine & Clinical Hospital Center Zagreb, Zagreb, (Croatia)+++; telmed@mef.hr
Kovač	M	Professor/ BSEE	Faculty of Electrical Engineering and Computing, University of Zagreb, Telemedicine Committee-Ministry of Health and Social Welfare (Member); Croatian Telemedicine Society-Croatian Medical Association (Board Member), Zagreb (Croatia)+++; mario.kovac@fer.hr

Lam	D	MD, MPH	University of Maryland School of Medicine; National Study Center for Trauma and Emergency Medical Systems; U.S. Army Telemedicine and Advanced Technology Research Center (TATRC); NATO/COMEDS Telemedicine Panel (Secretary), Brussels (Belgium) +++; Lam@TATRC.ORG
Ljubičić	N	Professor/MD	Minister of Health and Sociel Welfare, Croatian Government, Zagreb (Croatia) +++; neven.ljubicic@miz.hr
Lymberis	A	Mr.	European Commission, IST Directorate, Brussels, (Belgium) +; andreas.lymberis@cec.eu.int
Miličić	D	Professor/MD	Department of Cardiology, Zagreb Clinical Hospital Center; Croatian Society of Cardiology (President); Croatian Telemedicine Society, Zagreb (Vice-president); Telemedicine Committee-Ministry of Health and Social Welfare (Vice President) Zagreb (Croatia)+++; d.milicic@mail.inet.hr
Mittermayer	R	MD	Ministry of Health and Social Welfare (Deputy/Minister); Telemedicine Committee-Ministry of Health and Social Welfare (Member), Zagreb (Croatia)+++; renato.mittermayer@miz.hr
Noć	M	Professor/MD	Department of Cardiology, University of Ljubljana, (Slovenia) +++
Oto	A	Professor/MD	Turkish Society of Cardiology (President), Ankara (Turkey)++
Parkromenko	AN	Professor/MD	Institute of Cardiology, Kyiv (Ukraine)++
Pavelin	A	BSEE	T-Com Service Department, Business Services and Solutions, Zagreb (Croatia) +++; Aljosa.Pavelin@t.ht.hr
Poropatich	R	COL/MD/ Professor	US Army Medical Research & Materiel Command; Telemedicine and Advanced Technology Research Center, Fort Detrick, MD (USA) +++; Ron.Poropatich@DET.AMEDD.ARMY.MIL
Primorac	D	Professor/MD	Minister of Science, Education and Sports, Croatian Government, Zagreb (Croatia)+++; ministar@mzos.hr
Racoceanu	CR	MD	INFO World, Bucharest (Romania) +++; cristina.racoceanu@infoworld.ro

Rončević	B		Minister of Defence, Croatian Government, Zagreb (Croatia)+++; infor@morh.hr
Rudowski	R	MD	Department of Medical Informatics and Telemedicine, Medical University of Warsaw (Poland) +++; rrudowsk@amwaw.edu.pl
Šimunović	Pjer	Professor	Ministry of Foreign Affairs, Coordinator for NATO, Zagreb, (Croatia)+++; pjer.simunovic@mvp.hr
Stamati	A	Professor/MD	Institute of Cardiology (Moldova)+++; adela@ch.moldpac.md
Vardas	P	Professor MD	Department of Cardiology, University of Krete (Greece); European Society of Cardiology (Vice President) ++
Van Hoof	R	Major General/MD	NATO COMEDS (Chairman), Brussels (Belgium) roger.vanhoof@mil.be +++
Vulić	S	PhD	Ministry of Health and Social Welfare, Zagreb (Croatia); IBRD Loan-Project Program (Director), Zagreb (Croatia)+++ spaso.vulic@miz.hr
Walderhaug	S	Engineer	S.P. Andersensv. 15B, 7465 Trondheim (Norway)+++; stale.walderhaug@sintef.no

Participants

Surname	Initials	Title	Institute
Adilova	FT	Professor	National Coordinator on Telemedicine, National Academy of Sciences, Inst. Of Informatics (Uzbekistan) +++ fatima_adilova@rambler.ru; fatima_adilova@ic.uz
Chevalier	MC	MD	HIA Robert Picque, Bordeaux (France) +
Čikeš	I	Professor/MD	Croatian Academy of Sciences, Zagreb (Member); Department of Cardiology, Zagreb Clinical Hospital Center, Zagreb (Head) (Croatia) +++; icikes@rebro.mef.hr
Duvančić	S	MD	Ministry of Defence, Croatian Government, Zagreb (Croatia) +++; sduvanci@morh.hr
Grabowski	M	MD	Cardiology Clinic, 1st Faculty of Medicine, Medical University of Warsaw, Warsow (Poland) +++; rrudowsk@amwaw.edu.pl

Ilinca	G	MD	INFO World, Bucharest (Romania) +++; cristina.racoceanu@infoworld.ro
Katić	M	Professor/MD	Zagreb University School of Medicine; Department of Family Medicine, School of Public Health "Andrija Štampar", Zagreb (Croatia) +++; milica.katic@mef.hr
Szymanski	F	MD	Cardiology Clinic, 1st Faculty of Medicine, Medical University of Warsaw (Poland) +++; rrudowsk@amwaw.edu.pl
Sagen	T	Lieutenant Colonel	Ministry of Defense, Oslo (Norway) +++
Sierdzinski	J	Professor	Department of Medical Informatics and Telemedicine, Medical University of Warsaw (Poland) +++; rrudowsk@amwaw.edu.pl
Stevanović	R	Professor/MD	Croatian Institute of Public Health, Zagreb (Croatia) +++; ranko.stevanovic@hzjz.hr

VIP Participants

Surname	Initials	Title	Institute
Čikeš	N	Professor/MD	Dean, Zagreb University School of Medicine, Zagreb (Croatia) +++; nada.cikes@mef.hr
Ćosić	K	General/ Professor/ BSEE	Representative, Parliament of Croatia, University of Zagreb, Faculty of Electrical Engineering and Computing Zagreb (Croatia) +++; kresimir.cosic@fer.hr
Dachev	TP	PhD	Bulgarian Academy of Sciences (Member), Sofia (Bulgaria) +++; tdachev@bas.bg
Golem	AZ	MD	State Secretary, Ministry of Health and Social Welfare, Zagreb (Croatia) +++; antezvonimir.golem@mzss.hr
Kos	M	Professor/ BSEE	Dean, Faculty of Electrical Engineering and Computing, Zagreb (Croatia) +++; mladen.kos@fer.hr
Lievens	F	Mr.	Board Member and Treasurer, International Society for Telemedicine-e Health (IsfTeH), Brussels (Belgium) +++; lievens@skynet.be
Lucić	J	General	Chief of Staff, Croatian Army, Zagreb (Croatia)+++; infor@morh.hr

Morau	A	CPT/MD	Minister, Ministry of National Defense, Medical Directorate, 3–5 Strada Institutul Medico Militar, Bucharest (Romania) +++; MORARUA@RO.PIMS.ORG
Muja	S	MD	Telemedicine Association of Kosovo, Zone "Ulpiana" No. 45, Prishtine (Kosovo) +++; sh_muja@yahoo.com
Rajner	Ž	Professor/MD	President, Croatian Academy of Medical Sciences; Head, Zagreb Clinical Hospital Center, Zagreb (Croatia) +++; zeljko.rajner@rebro.mef.hr
Raos	P	Professor	President, Telemedicine Association Zagreb; Vice-president, Croatian Telemedicine Society, Zagreb (Croatia) +++; praos@public.srce.hr
Raboteg	M	CSEE	State Secretary, Ministry of Defence, Zagreb (Croatia)+++; infor@morh.hr
Schwarz	D	MD	Deputy/Minister, Ministry of Science, Education and Sports, Croatian Government, Zagreb (Croatia) +++; dragan.schwarz@mzos.hr
Šostar	Z	MD	Head, City Office for Health, Labor and Social Welfare, City of Zagreb; Healthy City Project Coordinator (Croatia) +++; zvonimir.sostar@zagreb.hr

Index

E. Telecardiology for rural areas: Bulgarian experience

Malina Jordanova

Institute of Psychology, Bulgarian Academy of Sciences, Sofia, Bulgaria

F. Advanced Technology: Research, application and integration of 3D structural information with multimedia contents for tele-virtual Dg./therapy: possible use in the NATO environment

Ivica Klapan [a,b,c]
Ljubimko Šimičić [c]
Sven Lončarić [d,e]
Mario Kovač [d]
Ante-Zvonimir Golem [b,c,f]
Juraj Lukinović [a,b,c]

[a] University Department of ENT, Head & Neck Surgery, Division of Plastic and Reconstructive Head & Neck Surgery and Rhinosinusology, Zagreb University School of Medicine, Salata 4, Zagreb, Croatia
[b] Zagreb University Hospital Center, Zagreb, Croatia
[c] Reference Center for Computer Aided Surgery and Telesurgery, Ministry of Health, Republic of Croatia, Zagreb, Croatia
[d] Faculty of Electrical Engineering and Computing, University of Zagreb, Croatia
[e] Department of Electrical and Computer Engineering, New Jersey Institute of Technology, Newark, USA
[f] Ministry of Health and Social Welfare Republic of Croatia

G. ICT in telemedicine/telecardiology system on Croatian islands: the potential utility of this technology on a regional basis in the south-eastern Europe

Mario Kovač [a]
Ivica Klapan [b,c,d]

[a] Faculty of Electrical Engineering and Computing, University of Zagreb, Croatia
[b] University Department of ENT, Head & Neck Surgery, Division of Plastic and Reconstructive Head & Neck Surgery and Rhinosinusology, Salata 4, Zagreb University School of Medicine
[c] Zagreb University Hospital Center, Zagreb, Croatia
[d] Reference Center for Computer Aided Surgery and Telesurgery, Ministry of Health, Salata 4, Zagreb, Croatia

H. The future isn't what it used to be—Applying new technologies in health care

David Lam [a]
Ronald Poropatich [b]

[a] U.S. Army Telemedicine and Advanced Technology Research Center, Ft. Detrick Maryland and University of Maryland School of Medicine, National Study Center for Trauma and Emergency Medical Services, Baltimore, Maryland
[b] U.S. Army Telemedicine and Advanced Technology Research Center, Ft. Detrick Maryland

I. PacRim pediatric heartsounds trial: store-and-forward pediatric telecardiology evaluation with echocardiographic validation

MAJ C. Becket Mahnke
LTC Michael P. Mulreany

Medical Corps, U.S. Army
Tripler Army Medical Center
Pediatric Dept., Honolulu, HI

J. Remote controlled robot performing real-time echocardiography on distance – a new possibility in emergency and dangerous areas

Mona Olofsson [a,b]
Kurt Boman [a,b,c]

[a] Department of Medicine, Skellefteå County Hospital
[b] HeartNet, Skeria, Skellefteå
[c] Department of Public Health and Clinical Medicine, Umeå University, Sweden

K. A functional telemedicine environment in the framework of the Croatian healthcare information system

Pavelin Aljoša [b,e]
Klapan Ivica [a,b,d]
Kovač Mario [a,b,d]
Katić Milica [b,c,f]
Stevanović Ranko [b,g]
Rakić Mladen [b,h]
Klapan Nives [i]

[a] Telemedicine Committee, Ministry of Health and Social Welfare, Republic of Croatia
[b] Croatian Telemedicine Society, Croatian Medical Association, Zagreb, Croatia
[c] Committee for development of State program of health care and development of telemedicine on islands, Ministry of the Sea, Tourism, Transport and Development, Republic of Croatia

[d] Reference center of the Ministry of Health and Social Welfare for computerized surgery and telesurgery, Zagreb, Croatia
[e] Metronet telekomunikacije d.d, Sektor za mrežu i usluge, Zagreb, Croatia
[f] Department of Family Medicine, School of Public Health «Andrija Štampar», Zagreb, Croatia
[g] Croatian Institute for Public Health, Zagreb, Croatia
[h] Clinical Hospital Split, Department of Anesthesiology and Intensive Care, Split, Croatia
[i] Department of Telemedicine, Zagreb, Croatia

L. Telemedicine standardization in the NATO environment

David Lam [a]
Ronald K. Poropatich [b]
Gary R.Gilbert [c]

[a] Charles McC. Mathias National Study Center for Trauma and Emergency Medical Systems, Baltimore Maryland, and U.S. Army Telemedicine and Advanced Technology Research Center, Fort Detrick Maryland
[b] Walter Reed Army Medical Center, Washington, D.C., and U.S. Army Telemedicine and Advanced Technology Research Center, Fort Detrick Maryland
[c] Department of Electrical Engineering, School of Engineering, University of Pittsburgh, Pittsburgh, PA, and U.S. Army Telemedicine and Advanced Technology Research Center, Fort Detrick Maryland

M. Redefining the future of healthcare through telecardiology and telemedicine

Cristina Racoceanu
George Ilinca

Infoworld
37–39, Intrarea Glucozei Street
2nd district, 023828
Bucharest, Romania

N. Telecardiological system for acute coronary syndromes in Mazovia district of Poland

Robert Rudowski[a]
Marcin Grabowski[a,b]
Janusz Sierdzinski[a]
Filip Szymanski[a,b]

[a] Department of Medical Informatics and Telemedicine, Medical University of Warsaw SP CSK Hospital, Banacha Str. 1A, 02-097 Warsaw, Poland
[b] Cardiology Clinic, 1-st Faculty of Medicine, Medical University of Warsaw

O. Development of diagnostic cardiology/telecardiology procedures in Republic of Moldova

Adela Stamati [a]
Mihail Popivici [b]

[a] Departement of pediatric cardiology, State Medical and Pharmaceutical University "Nicolae Testemitanu"; scientific secretary at Experts Council,
Minister of Health and Social Protection of Republic of Moldova
[b] Director of Institute of Cardiology, Republic of Moldova

P. Croatia and NATO

Aleksandar Sunko

Department for NATO, Political, Military and Security Issues
Republic of Croatia
Ministry of foreign affairs
1st political division for the European Union, NATO and member countries

Q. The future of the military medical services in NATO

Roger van Hoof

Major General, MD, Chairman COMEDS
Committee of the Chiefs of Military Medical Services in NATO
Secretariat: Department of Strategy
Headquarter Belgian Armed Forces
Everestreet 1, B 1140 Brussels, Belgium

R. Justification of investing in Telemedicine

Spase Vulić [a]
Nives Klapan [b]

[a] Program Director, The Ministry of Health and Social Welfare – Health System Project, Zagreb, Croatia
[b] Department of Telemedicine, Zagreb, Croatia

S. Telecardiology – patterns for current and future use

Ståle Walderhaug [a,b]
Per Håkon Meland [a]

[a] Research Scientist, Norwegian Joint Medical Service, MEDOPS/Ullevål University Hospital, OSLO MIL/Akershus, 0015 Oslo, Norway
[b] Research Scientist, SINTEF ICT, SP Andersensvei 15b, 7465 Trondheim, Norway

Contents

Remote Cardiology Consultations Using Advanced Medical Technology
I. Klapan and R. Poropatich (Eds.)
IOS Press, 2006

Spanish Military Telecardiology

Alberto Hernández ABADIA DE BARBARA[a], Enrique Selva BELLOD[b]

[a] *Telemedicine Unit. Hospital Central de la Defensa "Gómez Ulla".Inspección General de Sanidad del Ministerio de Defensa, Glorieta del Ejército s/n. 28047, Madrid. Spain*

[b] *Cardiology Department. Hospital Central de la Defensa "Gómez Ulla".Inspección General de Sanidad del Ministerio de Defensa,Madrid. Spain*

Abstract. This article describes the Spanish Military Telemedicine system and specially the role of the Telecardiology on it. Terrestrial wide area networks and satellite connections are used for cardiologic Teleconsultations and for clinical meetings. Coronariographies, ultrasound and the most of the cardiologic examinations are transmitted by these system. Some investigations on Telecardiology are on developing.

The paper was presented at the Advanced Research Workshop «Remote Cardiology Consultations Using Advanced Medical Technology – Applications for NATO Operations», held in Zagreb, Croatia 13-16 September 2005

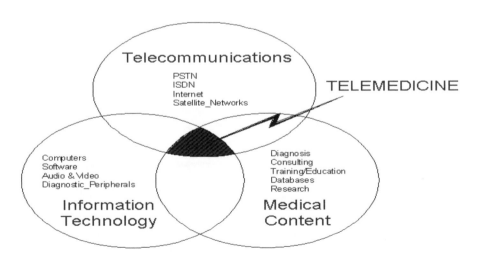

1. Spanish Military Telecardiology

The "American Medical Association" defines Telemedicine as "the provision of health-cares consultation and education, using Telecommunication Networks to communicate information".

Telemedicine is included within the area of eHealth. A Teleconsultation forms the main part of Telemedicine and usually is done between two medical providers, one who asks for special diagnostic or therapeutic advice, and the other one who provides it.

Undoubtedly Telemedicine is a very important tool for different Medical Corps which can use it in many different terrains and environments.

The Spanish Ministry of Defence (MoD) deployed its new Telemedicine system in February 2002. The aim of this was mainly to support Medical Treatment Facilities Role 2 - 2+ levels from the Army, the Navy and the Air Force deployed on different International Missions all around the world.

Medical Personnel are supported by the Directorate of the Medical Corp of the MoD (IGESAN). Modular Attendant Teams (MAT) are composed of one trauma surgeon, one anesthesiologist, one orthopedic surgeon, one critical care specialist and three nurse officers. These Role 2 units require at least one MAT from the beginning of deployment.

The Role 2 MTF (Medical Treatment Facility) is one of the units that can be supported through the use of a Telemedicine system. Our critical care specialists are trained for assessing and treating different acute cardiac diseases but a second opinion from a cardiologist is a valuable help that sometimes is needed. There are many other specialities that could be supported too, such as radiology, dermatology, psychiatry, internal medicine, and neurosurgery, and up to 15 Specialities on ward and 13 more on call 24/7.

A satellite connection is used for a communications link between the deployed units and the national military hospitals. Inmarsat technology is used for this purpose with a bandwidth of 128 Kbps, and the videoconference system applies videocodec H-264. This videoconference allows real time reception of echocardiography examinations that are carried out by an Intensivist who is deployed on an International Mission, and is assessed by a cardiologist in one of the different Military Hospitals in Spain.

The Spanish Military Telemedicine Reference Centre located in the Central Defence Hospital "Gómez Ulla" in Madrid maintains operability 24 hours due to Nurses Officers being on continual duty. These support the Specialist Medical Officers on ward that can be consulted at any moment, and the Telemedicine equipment is operated by these nurses while the Teleconsultations are being carried out.

From December 2003 all Spanish military hospitals have Telemedicine sets installed. This system interconnects eight hospitals via videoconference and facilitates real time transmission of radiology, digital images, vital signs real time and multiconference. The eight Spanish military hospitals and the infirmaries of some military bases are integrated in a private Wide Area Network (WAN) with 1 Mb of bandwidth. Together both kinds of connections (satellite and dedicated terrestrial network) constitute the Spanish Military Telemedicine Network.

These Telemedicine settings give military medical treatment facilities the following capabilities:

- Real time videoconference.
- Visual examinations.
- Diagnostic imaging: X-Ray pictures, teleultrasound examination, CT scan, MRI…. All of them can be generated physically (scanned and digitalized later) or digital format.
- Vital signs transmission in real time: telemonitoring of cardiac frequency, NIBP, SpO2 and temperature.

Currently there are Telemedicine sets on the three Role 2+ Army units, 6 Navy ships and the Role 2 Air force MTF units as well as the Aeromedical Evacuation Unit.

All of them connect with the Military Hospital net via Inmarsat.

The main Telemedicine Unit of this WAN is located in the Hospital Central de la Defensa "Gómez Ulla" that is situated in Madrid. This Unit has one Reference Center where Teleconsultations are carried out.

There also exists a Telemedicine laboratory where a Telemedicine specialist oversees training with the different devices used for Teleconsultations (general examinations cameras, ultrasound machine, telemicroscope, etc).

Additionally there is one classroom for fifteen people, where lessons are taught or where some of the interactive clinical meetings of the Military Hospitals and other civilian institutions are coordinated. The Telemedicine Unit works also in a multifunctional room for 125 people and a larger one for 440 people.

All the MEDEVACs to the "Gómez Ulla" hospital have to be assessed on a previous Teleconsultation, with the aim of avoiding non indicated MEDEVACS and/or helping other professionals with recommendations about transportation and other measures to take in advance.

Clinical meetings with the Cardiology department, Intensive Care Unit and the Cardiac Surgery department are conducted (via Telemedicine) every Friday morning with the interactive attendant of personnel from the Military Hospitals and from other Medical Treatment Facilities.

There is going on one study about Teleauscultation on digital format with the application of telefonocardiography.

The Cardiology department and the Telemedicine Unit are working together on the application of 3G videoconference for Teleconsultations with patients and specialists located outside of the hospital.

References

[1]   Ferrer-Roca O, Sosa-Iudicissa M. Handbook of Telemedicine. Ámsterdam 1998.
[2]   Ferrer-Roca O. La Telemedicina: Situación actual y perspectivas. Fundación Retevisión. 2001. Madrid.
[3]   Luces y sombras de la información de salud en Internet. Informe Seis. Pamplona 18 de junio de 2002.
[4]   Alfaro Ferreres L, García Rojo M, Puras Gil A. Manual de Telepatología. Pamplona 2001.
[5]   Beolchi L. Telemedicine Glossary. European Commission. 2002 Working Document.
[6]   Sánchez-Caro J, Abellán F. Telemedicina y protección de datos sanitarios. Editorial Comares S.L. Granada 2002.
[7]   Tromso Telemedicine Conference. 15-17 September 2003. Tromso Norway.
[8]   Archivos de Telemedicina de Sanidad Militar. 1996-2003.
[9]   Lessons Learned in Telemedicine. 2000-2005. Telemedicine Panel. NATO.
[10] Zamorano J, Gil-Loyzaga P, Miravet D. Telemedicina: Análisis de la situación actual y perspectiva de futuro. Fundación Vodafone 2004. Madrid.

[11] González F, Zamarrón C. Telemedicina: Aplicaciones y nuevas tecnologías. Sociedad Gallega de Telemedicina. Santiago 2004.
[12] Klapan I, Cikeš I. Telemedicine. Telemedicine Association. Zagreb 2005.

Future Collaboration in Diagnostics and Follow-up of Patients with Acute Coronary Syndrome: Telecardiology Experience of Dubrava University Hospital, Zagreb, Croatia

Mijo BERGOVEC, Andreja PERSOLI
Dubrava University Hospital, Avenija G.Suska 6, Zagreb, Croatia

The paper was presented at the Advanced Research Workshop «Remote Cardiology Consultations Using Advanced Medical Technology – Applications for NATO Operations», held in Zagreb, Croatia 13-16 September 2005

1. Introduction

"Reperfusion therapy in acute coronary syndromes (ACS) is a milestone achievement in 20th century cardiology" (Braunwald E, 2004). This therapy includes thrombolysis, primary coronary angioplasty (PCI) and stent implantation, and coronary artery bypass surgery (CABG) in patients with ST segment elevation in electrocardiogram in acute myocardial infarction. Immediate primary PCI (as soon as possible) from the beginning of the ACS is considered the best solution. In the case of immediate primary PCI, ischemic myocardial infarction, mortality and invalidity are significantly reduced, recovery time is shortened, and quality of patient's life is improved.

It is very important to shorten the time of medical intervention for reperfusion therapy at any level of medical care: symptoms recognition, calling to medical system, prehospital recognition of a problem including electrocardiographic recording and therapy beginning, transport to hospital, and transport into laboratory for coronary interventions. Delay in initiation of reperfusion therapy increases loss of myocites at any level from beginning of symptoms to catheter laboratory.

"Reperfusion therapy for acute myocardial infarction with ST elevation is a milestone achievement in 20th century cardiology"

2. Prehospital Procedures

According to the latest studies (DANAMI II, PRAGUE II, etc.), immediate transport to hospital with the primary PCI facilities is the best way for rapid restoration of blood flow in the infarct-related coronary artery.

European Society of Cardiology (ESC) and American Heart Association and American College of Cardiology (AHA/ACC) guidelines for prehospital procedure determine that patients with STEMI must be transferred to a tertiary center for primary PCI. If the patient is hospitalized into the medical center without reperfusion therapy option, the time spent until his transfer to tertiary center must be less than 90 minutes.

The goal is: 30 minutes for "door to needle" (the time from the arrival of medical personnel to fibrinolytic therapy administration), and 90 minutes for "door to balloon" (the time from the arrival of medical personnel to primary PCI). Loosing time at any level (symptoms recognition, alerting Emergency, prehospital medical personnel activation, setting diagnosis, transfer, admission in hospital, PCI facility and an experienced team activation) delay reperfusion time, and increases infarct size and mortality.

The main element in prehospital ACS diagnosis is the 12-lead ECG. Ambulance personnel should be trained to recognize the symptoms of ACS. It is desirable for ambulance staff to have a ECG device for diagnostic purposes even in patient's home, in the outdoors or in the Emergency vehicle. In the case of ACS diagnosis (or nonspecific findings), recorded ECG (from ECG-defibrillator monitor) should be sent to Coronary unity by mobile phone signal (telemedicine).

Guidelines of ESC and AHA/ACC suggest the following: "patients with STEMI should be brought immediately or secondarily transferred promptly (primary-receiving hospital door-to-departure time less than 90 minutes) to facilities capable of cardiac catheterization and rapid revascularization".

The usage of telemedicine in the prehospital care of the patient with ACS can significantly shorten the time from the moment of appearance of symptoms to primary PCI. The goal is to determine the right diagnoses and the ACS form with telemedicine methods, and after distinguishing risk factors to safely transfer patient to Clinical hospital for emergency cardiologic procedure.

Good communication between emergency medicine teams and referring hospital is "the must" in confirming diagnoses and beginning the right treatment of patient with ACS.

3.Emergency Ambulance Personnel in the Outdoors and Cardiology Specialist in PCI Center Communication

Emergency ambulance personnel in the outdoors, non-PCI and PCI center have following communication possibilities:
1. direct phone contact
2. sending ECG to non-PCI or PCI center by fax
3. cardiotelemedicine, with safe systems

In Dubrava University Hospital experience, communication between emergency medicine and cardiology department in PCI hospital is established by LIFENET system (Medtronic). LIFENET system consists of ECG defibrillator monitor, which sends 12-lead ECG (during the recording) through mobile phone to receiving station in non-PCI center, and if needed to PCI center (or directly to PCI center). Besides ECG other patient data is sent by the system (blood pressure, heart rate, oxygen saturation, used drugs etc.).

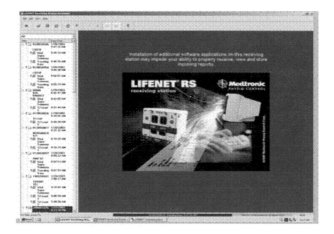

Figure 1. ECG transmission

In the moment of transmitting data alarm sounds in the receiving station in CCU, after which a cardiology specialist on call, after analyzing received data, can phone medical personnel who has sent the data.

In the case of ACS, patient must be transferred to a PCI center as soon as possible. During transport patient is monitored continuously.

If needed, medical staff by the patient side can contact the cardiology specialist at any time by mobile phone. Cardiology specialist, having the same data as medical personnel in the Emergency vehicle, can help his colleagues and if necessary correct the therapy or recognize life-threatening arhythmia.

This communication establishes the best way to set the right diagnoses, and what is most important, sets indication for primary invasive cardiology procedure even during the time when the patient is on the way to hospital. Invasive cardiology team, which is on call 24 hours a day, can get ready for the procedure, and save a lot of time, what is the main goal according to the 'time is muscle' dogma.

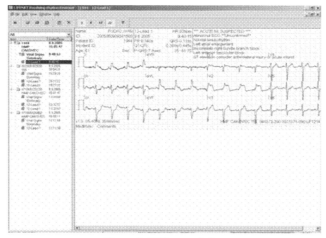

Figure 2. ECG transmission

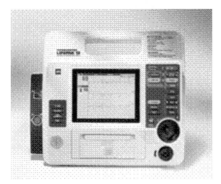
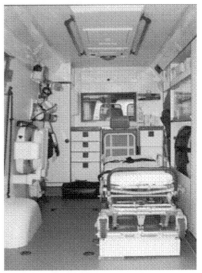

Figure 3 and 4. Equipment of EMS for fast patient transport with STEMI

4. Cardiotelemedicine Equipment in the Prehospital Teams

Sophisticated technology in this approach helps not only by safe and in time recognition of life-threatening conditions in the prehospital setting, but also by immediate mobilization of medical teams suitable for patient treatment. Besides, it allows data storage and/or wireless data transfer.

Emergency medicine teams should have all the equipment for life support in the Emergency vehicle, according to ACLS guidelines. The most important are compatible ECG defibrillator monitors with data transfer option (telemedicine). These vehicles are precondition "sine qua non" for cardiotelemedicine. The other precondition is a continuous controlled medical personnel education (emergency teams in the outdoors, personnel in non-PCI centers with receiving station, and personnel in PCI centers).

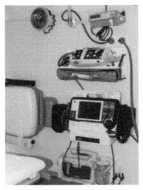
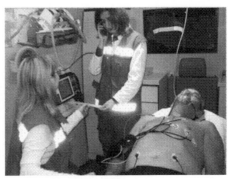

Figures 5 and 6. Equipment of EMS for fast patient transport with STEMI
and consultation by phone with cardiologist on duty

The last, but not the least precondition is a receiving station in hospitals compatible with the equipment outside the hospital.
Telemedicine allows:
- fast and safe transport from country to hospital,
- fast line to Emergency Department,
- fast direct line to invasive cardiac laboratory, and
- fast primary PCI.

5. Telemedicine in Croatia - What Have We Done?

Croatian Cardiac Society and Ministry of Health of the Republic of Croatia initiate the project "Primary PCI for STEMI patients in 3 hospitals in Zagreb from county centers" which comprises patients with STEMI in the ring of 120 km surrounding Zagreb: territory of county hospitals in towns Zagreb, Karlovac, Sisak, Zabok, Varazdin, Koprivnica, Bjelovar, and Cakovec. Regional centers Koprivnica, Bjelovar, and Cakovec are also assigned to Dubrava University Hospital.
Croatian Cardiac Society and Ministry of Health of Republic Croatia
County hospitals in ring 120 km surrounding Zagreb
Project: primary PCI for STEMI patients in 3 hospitals in Zagreb

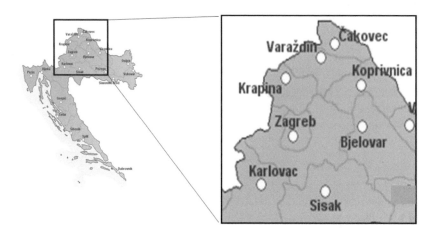

Figure 7. Croatian Cardiac Society and Ministry of Health of Republic Croatia

6. "Vrbovec Heart Safe Community" - the First Step of Cardiotelemedicine for Acute Coronary Syndromes in Croatia. Pilot Project

In the implementation of the project of Croatian Cardiac Society and Ministry of Health of the Republic of Croatia, the town of Vrbovec was the first step.

Vrbovec is the town on the east part of the county of Zagreb, with the population of 29,520 including its surroundings. Medical facility for primary medical care and a part of the specialists medical care is Branch Vrbovec Health centre county of Zagreb. The whole area gravitates towards Zagreb and all the patients are being transported to Dubrava University Hospital.

Department for cardiovascular diseases Dubrava University Hospital and Vrbovec Emergency closely cooperate in order to improve medical care for patients with life-threatening cardiovascular diseases. Project has been named "Vrbovec Heart safe community". Agreement between these two institutions has been signed, and the Protocol for patient care with ACS from county of Vrbovec has been made. Protocol defines exact obligations and general responsibilities in the cardiac patient care for both institutions. One of the established proceedings is telemedicine's 12-lead ECG transmission with LIFENET system.

Equipment for Emergency units in Vrbovec has been provided. Continuous education includes ERC courses: BLS-AED course, ACLS course, "ECG in medical practice", active participation in Croatian and international scientific meetings and congresses, and regular practical training.

Except Emergency teams, who are directly involved, 17 general practice physicians in county of Vrbovec also take part in the project. For the large area (520 km2), health care has been provided in 8 medical centres. Each centre has been equipped with AED, compatible with the equipment in the Emergency vehicle, which allows data transfer. Physicians and other medical personnel has been involved in emergency medical care and life support education.

In the year 2003, Dubrava University Hospital and Emergency medical unit Vrbovec were provided with the appropriate telemedicine equipment and have received necessary education for treating the patients involved in telemedicine.

Emergency medical unit Vrbovec is the pioneer of telemedicine in ACS in Croatia. With the introduction of new technology, education of medical personnel and laymen, and with media support of this project, Vrbovec has established guidelines for other "Heart safe communities".

Summary of telecardiology in acute coronary syndromes in Vrbovec community:
- June 15th, 2004 to September 10th, 2005:
- 14 patients
- onset of symptoms to EMS call: 45 +/- 20 min
- onset of symptoms to first telecardiology ECG: 60+/- 35 min
- transport from Vrbovec to Dubrava hospital: 20 +/- 15 min
- time from onset of symptoms to PCI (balloon + stent): 125 +/- 45 min

7. Cardiotelemedicine in the County of Medjimurje - The Second Step

According to the Pilot project "Vrbovec Heart safe community", the same education was performed in the county of Medjimurje. Doctors and nurses from emergency service and county of Medjimurje Cakovec hospital with colleagues cardiologists from Dubrava University Hospital performed:
- basic life support and advanced life support courses,
- course "ECG in medical practice" for physicians,
- active participation in Croatian and international symposiums on emergency medicine and telemedicine,
- practical training, and
- education of population - media, seminars, lectures.

Example:
- pt: SS, male, age: 52
- onset of symptoms: June 12, 2005; time: 12:11
- place: Sv. Martin na Muri, county of Medjimurje, 19 km from Cakovec hospital
- call to EMS: 12.45
- first ECG: 13.05 transmission to Cakovec county hospital
- ECG sent to Dubrava University Hospital: 13:20
- PCI team - on place
- transport from Sv. Martin na Muri to Dubrava University Hospital (102 km) 13:30-14:25
- first needle: 14:35
- PCI balloon: 14:45
- PCI stent: 14:55
- time from onset of symptoms to PCI (balloon + stent): 164 minutes

Summary of telecardiology in STEMI patients in Dubrava University Hospital - county of Medjimurje:
- period: June 10th to September 10th, 2005:
- 13 patients
- onset of symptoms to EMS call: 35 +/- 25 min
- onset of symptoms to first telecardiology ECG: 48 +/- 30 min
- transport from Medjimurje to Dubrava hospital: 61 +/- 15 min
- time from onset of symptoms to PCI (balloon + stent): 144 +/- 40 min

Remote Cardiology Consultations Using Advanced Medical Technology
I. Klapan and R. Poropatich (Eds.)
IOS Press, 2006

The Use of Advance Medical Technologies in Telemedicine/ Telecardiology: Future Application and Design

Lorenco DAMJANIĆ

Ericsson Communication Software R&D (Shanghai) Co., Ltd., Shanghai

Abstract. This article is summarising trend and technologies which might be usefule for establishment of differen solution aplicable in area of Telemedicine/Telecardiology.Additionally some working assumption and support definitions are presented to be able to outline a possible integration strategy of telemedicine solution within a trully intrgrated information technology system what is an ultimate goal of every leading heath care organisation.

The paper was presented at the Advanced Research Workshop «Remote Cardiology Consultations Using Advanced Medical Technology – Applications for NATO Operations», held in Zagreb, Croatia 13-16 September 2005

1. Introduction

Adopting an definition for vertical market as a group of business, organisation or enterprice which are viewed as a clasification of the larger group of all businesses, organisations or enterprices on the base of the unique and specific nature of the products or services that they sell to the markets of the world or of the activities in

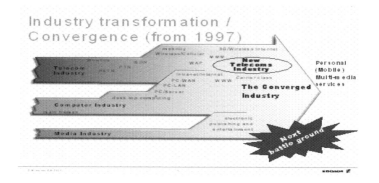

Figure 1.

Bit rates & Coverage for Wireless Technologies

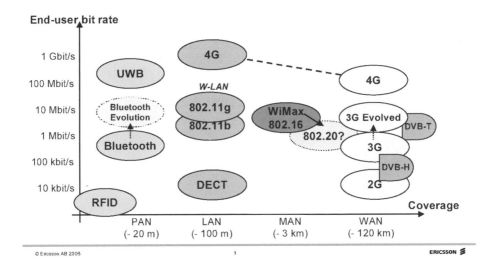

Figure 2.

which they are engaged lead us to the healtcare industry as one example of vertical market which main task is to prevent treat and mange of illness and preserv a mental and physical well/being trough the servicees offeres by the medical and allied health professions.

Using a vertical strategy for an IT vendor involves changing the whole approach to the market from a product-centred one to a demand-centred one. This requires in-depth analysis of IT spending patterns and of the forces that generate them in various industry sectors.

Although the healthcare industry is one of the world's largest and fastest-growing industry consuming over 10% of GDP for most developed country due to the fact that healthcare is a publicly-funded sector in most of Europe, limited funding may hamper fast growth in new projects.

For all these reason and ongoing convergence process towards new telecom industry (see figure 1) there are a lot of opportunities in the areas of content and collaborative solutions, managed services, and network infrastructure to enhance communication between patients, healthcare providers and healthcare payers.

Telecom has many new long-term growth opportunities

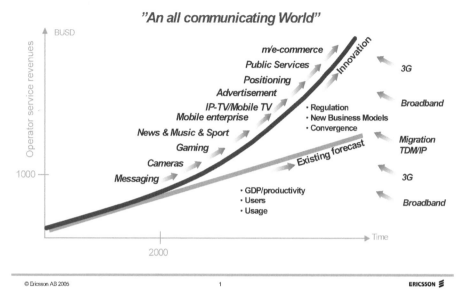

Figure 3.

1.1. Technological Trends

Considering continuos improvement in the access technology in fix as well as mobile area (see figure 2) follows by new business models and regulatory changes number of new services, which might be sources of operators revenues growh, dramaticaly changed existing forecast (see figure 3).

In parallel with these changes a process of end user device driven convergence (see figure 4) brings togethercompanies from differen industry segments (IT, telecom, ententiment) and most of the services become posible to be integrated in one device providing posibilities of mobile triple play enabling traditionaly home or office based serviced to be put on the mobile device. However a wireline access technology has chane from nerrowband to broadband technologies which brings possibilities of introducing two way broadband multi media applications at every and each home (see Figure 5).

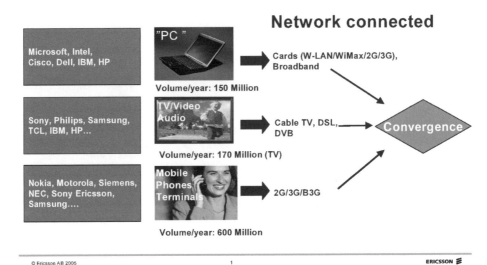

Figure 4.

Summaring all these technological/service trends an puting them in prospective of overall communication networks topology (see Figure 6), apart of core network which gredualy converge from circuite switch towards all IP (packet switch) technologies, different access networks are differenciated according to different access technology. For further discussion it is important to nouted thet Bluetooth technology is accounted for establisment of a personal area network (PAN) filling up an area of coverage person and a local area network (LAN).

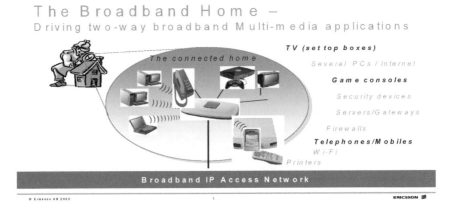

Figure 5.

1.2. Healthcare key business trends

The following are key trends for the healthcare market:

Patient safety – Different external groop have sdded preasure to the healthcare industry to reduce preventable patient errors. Providers have respondedby increasing ther efforts towards computer-base patient record (CPR) so the first Generation 3 CPR systems will emarhge soon.

Healthcare cost – Controlling the cost of health care is an ongoing problem and a key market force within both the payer and provider space. Heltcare benefits now constitute as high as 30 percent of total peyrole cost.

Collaboration – To support the need for greater patient safety and reduce cost, data is being shearing. This collaboration is not only between departments within the healthcare organisation; it is extending across to other healtcare organisations and down to the patient.

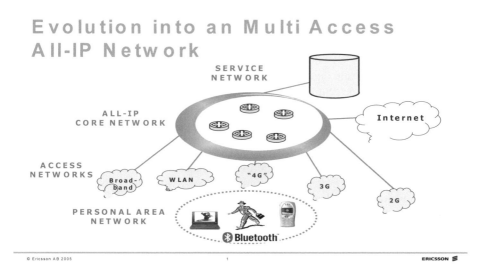

Figure 6.

2. Discussion

By defining Telemedicine as a generic term referring to all forms of medical information exchange by using a *variety of telecom technologies* to be able to provide medical expertise to places that due to their physical distance do not have access to this kind of competence which could be use as decision support for pre-hospital personnel working in ambulance or in patients` home as well as for transfer of important medical information from the remote location to a hospital or some other institution and using some of presented enabling telecom technology depends of a specific domain issue.

It is possible to develop number of telemedicine services such as: Tele consultancy, Ambulatory patient monitoring, Cardiac paging system, Remote treadmill stress testing, Monitoring in emergency department, Medical Transportation (air/land/sea).

To be able to successfully implement these applications there is a need for a strategic alliance between:

•Monitoring company that understand monitoring and

•Telecom provider that understand network system, wireless transitions, wireless System and paging to make reality wide spread implementation of system that has been designed to work within hospital or between remote user and hospital.

Once when the cooperation is established by ccombining multi parameter telemetry technology and digital video technology (videoconferencing) it is possible to establish a telemedicine centre, which could provide at least two distinct services:

-    remote telemedicine to rural hospital and clinics
-    telemedicine training (distance learning services).

One successfully example of this approach is a trial version of the Telemedicine Centre of the Ministry of Health Republic of Croatia.

Although telemedicine center address a substantial part of key trends within healthcare domain it is necessary to address rest of requirements that might be seen thought a vision of leading health care organization to have a *truly integrated information technology system*, which would allow it to provide access to patient records for personnel who required it regardless of where they are located.

Information systems need to be integrated across departments, platforms, applications, formats, geography, or strategy ally systems.

These systems are designed to meet the information needs of:

• Health enterprises,
• Public health institutions,
• Hospitals,
• Physicians
• Extended and residential care provider,
• Consumers,
Including:
• Clinical applications,
• Financial and administrative applications,
• Enterprise management applications,
• Decision support applications.

Still multi domain collaboration (technology vs. medical community) and multi vendor end to end integration would stay as very important facto to transform a trial telemedicine network to the full scale Telemedicine Center anticipating that full integration with a hospital information system is required.

3. Conclusion

Together with partners, especialy domain experts, Ericsson will be able to understend and satisfy the process needs of the healthcare players and implement trully inovative solution, applicable in the area of telemedicine/telecardiology, which would enrich the Ericsson's e-health product portafolio (www.ericsson.com/hr/products/e/health/index/shtml). Also it will be possible to contribute to cost reductions in healthcare and increas quality of life for patients.

References

[1] Report: WinterGreen Research, Laxington MA Healthcare Telecommunications – Telemedicine The Impact of the Internet, Integration Strategies, Market Strategies, Market Oportunities, Market Forecasts 2001-2006, www.wintergreenresearch.com

[2] Report: Berggren, M. Wireless communication in telemedicine using Bluetooth and IEEE 802.11b Department of Information Technology Uppsala University, TR 2001-208 November 2001 ISSN 1404-3203

[3] Article: Alping, A. &0 GHz Wireless- Applications, Technologies, and the SSF/HFE 60 GHz WLAN Project Proceedings of 60GHz Workshop 2001 15-16 May 2001 Onsala Herrgard, Kungsbacka, Sweden

[4] Presentation: Ericsson Internal Ericsson strategy-Global trends and local Markets

[5] Research Brief: Key Verticale Market trends Shape IT Initiative in 2005, January 2005, Marketplace code G00125629, www.gartner.com

[6] Forecast: Global industries, Worldwide 2002-2007, March 2004, www.gartner.com

[7] Book: Klapan,I., Čikeš, I.: Telemedicina u Hrvatskoj, Medika Zagreb 2001, ISBN 953-98509-2-4

Retrieved from: "http://en.wikipedia.org/wiki/Vertical_market

Telemedicine in the Context of Free Movement of Services in the EU: Legal and Policy Issues

Iris GOLDNER LANG

Faculty of Law, University of Zagreb, Trg Maršala Tita 14,
Zagreb, Croatia

Abstract. The paper addresses telemedicine, as a tool which enables better medical services to patients around the world, in its legal and policy context. In order for this new area of medicine to function properly, providing a safe, desirable and high-quality environment, technological developments should be followed, if not preceded, by legal and policy documents, thus avoiding any misuse, legal uncertainty and risks. The paper represents a screening exercise of the EU and Croatian legal and policy documents in this area and pinpoints problems and challenges faced today. The discussion shows not only where we are standing at this point, as regards legal and policy aspects of telemedicine in the EU and Croatia, but also suggests where we are heading and what our goals are. Any future developments in telemedicine require the establishment of all legal and policy preconditions for its safe practice.

The paper was presented at the Advanced Research Workshop «Remote Cardiology Consultations Using Advanced Medical Technology – Applications for NATO Operations», held in Zagreb, Croatia 13-16 September 2005

1. Introduction

Legal and policy issues in telemedicine have to be analyzed by, first, placing telemedicine into its legal habitat in the European Union (and in Croatia, as a candidate country that has started accession negotiations with the EU and is aspiring to join the Union in the years to come) – freedom to provide services, as one of the four fundamental freedoms of Community law. The definition of the freedom to provide services already reveals that telemedicine should be regarded as a service in the EU. It entails the carrying out of an economic activity for a temporary period in a Member State in which either the provider of the recipient of the service is not established.[1] The definition clarifies that four basic characteristics of services have to be fulfilled in order for Community law on services to apply: temporary character of the provision of services, the existence of a cross-border element, the service needs to be provided by a natural or a legal person and its provision has to be remunerated.

When it comes to the cross-border requirement, three situations can be envisaged. First, a service provider can be moving from his home Member State to another Member State where he temporarily provides services. This would be the case where the physician regularly practiced medicine in one Member State, but occasionally crossed the border with another Member State where he temporarily provided medical services to patients residing there. Second, a service recipient may be moving from his home Member State to another Member State for the purpose of receiving the service required. In this situation, the patient would be the one crossing the border in order to reach the physician. Significantly, neither of these two situations applies to telemedicine. Telemedicine can be placed in the third possible group of cases of the provision of services under Community law. This is the situation where neither the service provider, nor the service recipient moves, but it is the medical service itself that crosses the border between the two Member States.

Article 49 of the EC Treaty stipulates that "restrictions on freedom to provide services within the Community shall be prohibited in respect of nationals of Member States who are established in a State of the Community other than that of the person for whom the services are intended". This means that no discrimination is allowed towards service providers from other Member States who want to provide services in the host Member State, in comparison to domestic service providers. The respective provision, therefore, protects physicians who are providing medical services cross-border in the EU by the use of telemedicine, by banning any kind of discrimination in comparison to domestic service providers. Article 50 of the EC Treaty further elaborates that "services shall be considered to be "services" within the meaning of this Treaty where they are normally provided for remuneration, insofar as they are not governed by the provisions relating to freedom of goods, capital and persons" and continues by stating that "services shall in particular include: (a) activities of an industrial character; (b) activities of a commercial character; (c) activities of craftsmen; (d) activities of the professions".

2. EC Secondary Law Applicable to Telemedicine

So far telemedicine has been discussed in the context of EC primary law. On the other hand, EC secondary law applicable to telemedicine consists of a number of directives, not particularly aimed at telemedicine. Significantly, none of the legal documents mentioned below specifically addresses telemedicine, but covers a much wider area and, thus, encompasses telemedicine services. Directive 1997/7 on the protection of consumers in respect of distance contracts[2] and Directive 2000/31 on certain legal aspects of information society services in particular electronic commerce in the internal market (the so called "Directive on electronic commerce")[3] form the framework for telemedicine services. Directive on electronic commerce defines "information society services" as "any service normally provided for remuneration at a distance by electronic means at the individual request of a recipient of a service".[4] This definition is in line with the definition of services in general. The Directive furthermore stipulates that Member States may not "restrict the freedom to provide information society services from another Member State.[5] Measures that would derogate from the equal treatment principle can only be justified by reasons of public policy, public health, public security or the protection of consumers.[6] Prohibition of any kind of discrimination and the tolerated exceptions highly resemble EC Treaty provisions on services in general, as stipulated by Articles 49 and 55 of the EC Treaty. According to the established case-law of the European Court of Justice, public policy, public health and public security derogations should be interpreted narrowly, not allowing Member States any kind of misuse that would prevent or reduce cross-border movement.

Individual data protection in electronical communications, applicable also to the data processed in telemedicine, is regulated by two Directives. Directive 1995/46 on protection of individuals when processing personal data and on free movement of such data[7] provides for the right of privacy when personal data is processed. The second directive in this field is Directive 1997/66 on processing of personal data and protection on privacy in telecommunications sector.[8] Finally, Directive 93/42 concerning medical devices[9] establishes quality requirements standards and procedural measures prior to placing the equipment onto the internal market.

3. Guidelines for Practicing Telemedicine in the EU and Croatia

As stated previously, none of the EC secondary law applicable to telemedicine specifically addresses telemedicine *per se*, but covers a much wider range of issues that also encompass telemedicine. Therefore, when searching for specific documents on telemedicine both in Croatia and in the EU, only the following legally non-binding documents could be identified. In Croatia, the Telemedicine Committee of Croatian Ministry of Health, at its meeting on 15 March 2004 adopted "Croatian Telemedicine Strategy". The Strategy is a legally non-binding document completely based on the Standing Committee of European Doctors (CPME) Guidelines for Telemedicine. This means that most of the issues that will be mentioned below relating to the CPME Guidelines for Telemedicine, apply also to Croatian Telemedicine Strategy. Due to the fact that the members of the CPME are the EU Member States and some other states, such as Norway, the Guidelines are an important document throughout the EU. Although neither the CPME Guidelines for Telemedicine, nor Croatian Telemedicine Strategy are legally binding documents, their value should not be underestimated, since they have been developed by medical authorities and in some countries, such as Croatia, they serve as a professional norm that has to be followed.

The Guidelines consist of three parts: Ethical Guidelines in Telemedicine, Good Practice Guide for Marketing Professional Medical Services over the Net and CPME Guidelines for E-mail Correspondence in Patient Care. Ethical Guidelines in Telemedicine raise the issue of the state of authorization of physicians. In a physician-physician relation this is the state in which the physicians are located. On the other hand, in a physician-patient relation this is the state where the patient is normally resident or the service must be internationally approved. This brings us to the issue of the recognition of qualifications. Unless qualifications of physicians providing telemedicine services cross-border are recognized by the host Member State, in which the service is provided, the whole concept of the freedom of movement of services would be pointless and practically not functioning. Directive 93/16 to facilitate the free movement of doctors and the mutual recognition of their diplomas, certificates and other evidence of formal qualifications,[10] establishes the procedure of the recognition of physician's qualifications in EU Member States.[11] Although the Directive expressly covers only situations where the physician is moving cross-border and does not mention situations in which the service itself is moving, according to the established CPME policy the Directive should be understood as meaning that the physicians who are authorized to practice medicine in one Member State can provide telemedicine services cross-border in other EU Member States without further authorization. Another problem associated with the issue of the state of authorization of physicians is the recognition of medical prescriptions. In order to enable free movement of telemedicine services across the Union, a prescription of a doctor who is authorized to prescribe in one Member State should be valid in all other EU Member States.

The issue of the responsibility of treatment is another topic discussed by the Ethical Guidelines in Telemedicine. According to the Guidelines, in a physician-physician relation the responsibility lies with the physician asking for advice. Croatian Telemedicine Strategy furthermore extends the responsibility to the physician giving the advice, in case of his serious mistreatment. In a physician-patient relation the responsibility, naturally, lies with the physician involved in the case, while in case where a physician is performing medical interventions via telemedical techniques, he is the one being responsible.

The CPME Good Practice Guide for Marketing Professional Medical Services over the Net is another important part of the CPME Guidelines for Telemedicine. As its name clearly states, the Guide is applicable to marketing of professional medical services over the net, whether in the form of web-sites or by use of other display models. It is based on the principles set by Directive 200/31 (Directive on electronic commerce), which had to be transposed into Member States' national legal systems by 17 January 2002. The Directive promotes the use of commercial communications subject to "compliance with professional rules regarding, in particular, the independence, dignity and honor of the profession, professional secrecy and fairness towards clients and other members of the profession"[12] and obliges the Member States and the Commission to encourage "professional associations and bodies to establish codes of conduct at Community level",[13] which are in conformity with such professional rules. Following the cited provision of Directive 2000/31, the CPME has recommended to national medical associations to implement the Good Practice Guide for Marketing Professional Medical Services over the Net in the rules of the association or national regulations. Despite not being a CPME member, Croatian Telemedicine Committee of Croatian Ministry of Health has also followed the recommendation by including the Guide into Croatian Telemedicine Strategy.

Last, but not the least, the CPME Guidelines for E-mail Correspondence in Patient Care, emphasizes the importance of e-mail correspondence between a physician and a patient, which leaves behind a written document and thus increases legal certainty and the protection of both parties. However, one should take into consideration a number of legal risks of e-mail usage related to cross-border practice of telemedicine. First is the issue of jurisdiction in such situations. In the EU, this matter has been regulated by Regulation 2001/44 on jurisdiction and the recognition and enforcement of judgments in civil and commercial matters.[14] The Regulation basically leaves the choice of the court with the consumer, i.e. the patient. It allows the consumer to bring proceedings against the other party to a contract in the domicile of the consumer or in the domicile of the defendant, when the contract has been concluded in the domicile of the consumer or when the other party directs his professional activities to that Member State and the contract falls within the scope of such activities.[15] According to Croatian laws, the situation in Croatia can be slightly different, meaning that Croatian courts have jurisdiction when the defendant has residence in Croatia.

Another problem that might arise in case of cross-border practice of telemedicine is the issue of liability insurance coverage that protects the physician from financial losses if sued or condemned for liability. Finally, another matter that can cause problems in cross-border situations is the issue of reimbursement of telemedicine, i.e. health care insurance. Even though the EU does not have competence over health care systems and social security systems in Member States, the European Court of Justice has ruled that, with certain limitations, a patient can obtain out-patient and hospital care from another EU Member State and be reimbursed without prior permission by his sickness fund.[16]

4. Concluding Remarks

On 16 March 2002 the CPME adopted its policy entitled "The Practice of Telemedicine in Europe: Analysis, Problems and CPME Recommendations". The considerations and challenges that can be identified both from this document and the practice of telemedicine in the EU in general can be grouped as follows. First, the practice of telemedicine is still facing a number of gaps in legislation. Second, the existing general legislation on health care is not always sufficient for safe, high-quality practice of telemedicine. Third, there is still a certain degree of legal uncertainty for doctors and patients involved in cross-border practice of telemedicine. Finally, although the guidelines developed by international organizations are of extreme value for the development of telemedicine, one should not forget that they remain legally non-binding measures and, as such, could be less effective.

What can be done to overcome the outlined difficulties? Obviously, further encouragement of safe cross-border practice of telemedicine will require additional legislation to cover the existing gaps and control certain aspects of telemedicine. Second, one should continue developing and adopting further non-legislative measures, such as guidelines, which do have an important added value since they are in certain states respected by medical supervising authorities as professional norms that have to be followed. Finally, telemedicine *per se* could not exist without international cooperation in the regulative framework, which should be continued and strengthened.

References

[1]   Craig P, de Burca G. *EU Law – Text, Cases and Materials*. Oxford University Press, 2003: 800.
[2]   Directive 97/7/EC of the European Parliament and of the Council of 20 May 1997 on the protection of consumers in respect of distance contracts, OJ 1997, L 144.
[3]   Directive 2000/31/EC of the European Parliament and of the Council of 8 June 2000 on certain legal aspects of information society services, in particular electronic commerce, in the Internal Market ('Directive on electronic commerce'), OJ 2000, L 178.
[4]   Article 2(a) of the Directive on electronic commerce.

[5]   Article 3 of the Directive on electronic commerce.
[6]   Article 4(a)(i) of the Directive on electronic commerce.
[7]   Directive 95/46/EC of the European Parliament and of the Council of 24 October 1995 on the protection of individuals with regard to the processing of personal data and on the free movement of such data, OJ *1995,* L 281.
[8]   Directive 97/66/EC of the European Parliament and of the Council of 15 December 1997 concerning the processing of personal data and the protection of privacy in the telecommunications sector, OJ 1998, L 024.
[9]   Council Directive 93/42/EEC of 14 June 1993 concerning medical devices, OJ 1993, L 169.
[10] Council Directive 93/16/EEC of 5 April 1993 to facilitate the free movement of doctors and the mutual recognition of their diplomas, certificates and other evidence of formal qualifications, OJ 1993, L 165.
[11] Directive 93/16 will no longer be valid as of 20 October 2007, when it is to be replaced by the new Directive 2005/36/EC of the European Parliament and of the Council of 7 September 2005 on the recognition of professional qualifications, which has entered into force on 20 October 2005 and has to be transposed into the legal systems of the EU Member States by 20 October 2007.
[12] Article 8(1) of Directive 200/31 (Directive on electronic commerce): "Member States shall ensure that the use of commercial communications which are part of, or constitute, an information society service provided by a member of a regulated profession is permitted subject to compliance with the professional rules regarding, in particular, the independence, dignity and honor of the profession, professional secrecy and fairness towards clients and other members of the profession".
[13] Article 8(2) of Directive 200/31 (Directive on electronic commerce): "Without prejudice to the autonomy of professional bodies and associations, Member States and the Commission shall encourage professional associations and bodies to establish codes of conduct at Community level in order to determine the types of information that can be given for the purposes of commercial communication in conformity with the rules referred to in paragraph 1".
[14] Council Regulation (EC) No 44/2001 of 22 December 2000 on jurisdiction and the recognition and enforcement of judgments in civil and commercial matters, OJ 2001, L 012.
[15] Article 15 of Regulation 2001/44.
[16] Case C-158/96, *Kohll v. Union des Caisses de Maladie* [1998] ECR I-1931; Case C-120/95, *Decker* [1998] ECR I-1831; Case C-157/99, *Geraets-Smits v. Stichting Ziekenfonds, Peerbooms v. Stichting CZ Groep Zorgverzekeringen* [2001] ECR I-5473; Case C-368/98, *Vanbraekel v. ANMC* [2001] ECR I-5363.

Telecardiology for Rural Areas: Bulgarian Experience

Malina JORDANOVA

Institute of Psychology, Bulgarian Academy of Sciences, Sofia, Bulgaria

Abstract. The aim of this paper is to present in brief the attempts to develop a user-friendly environment for tele-cardiology consultations in a rural area as part of pilot project 7- BUL/03/001 co-funded by Bulgaria and International Telecommunication Union (ITU), Switzerland. The project is in its first half. The emphasis on tele-cardiology (monitoring and transmission of ECG, blood pressure and heart rate data) is due to the fact that cardiovascular diseases are leading cause of death in the country. The examination of vital cardiovascular parameters is the first and that's why the most often used tool providing clues to cardiovascular problems. Precise monitoring of these parameters is a good method to reveal first symptoms of coming myocardial infarct or other cardiovascular complications. Groups that will benefit from telecardiology application are patients suffering from cardiovascular diseases; patients on medications, which may affect the heart and elderly.

Acknowledgement:
The present study is conducted and will continue within next year in the context of the project 7- BUL/03/001 co-funded by Bulgaria and International Telecommunication Union (ITU), Switzerland and coordinated by Bulgarian Ministry of Transport and Communications.

The initial ideas of project 7- BUL/03/001 was presented at Med-e-Tel, Luxembourg, G.D. of Luxembourg, April 21-23, 2004.

The paper was presented at the Advanced Research Workshop «Remote Cardiology Consultations Using Advanced Medical Technology – Applications for NATO Operations», held in Zagreb, Croatia 13-16 September 2005.

1. Introduction

Telecardiology originates almost 35 years ago as a result of the necessity to monitor cardiovascular parameters of first group of patients with implanted pacemakers. This is the practice of cardiology utilizing state-of-the-art information and communication technologies. The aims of telecardiology are to provide chronically ill patients with access to specialized healthcare services as well as to increase the quality of their life by reducing the cost of treatment, reducing the inconvenience of traveling and periods of stay away from home and working environment.

Development of all aspects of telecardiology and its worldwide dissemination is a necessity because cardiovascular diseases are killer number 1 in Europe. They are not only the most common chronic diseases in Europe but they are also the most expensive diseases for healthcare providers. Today, it is impossible to list even the most outstanding publications in the area of telecardiology. They are thousands.

The aim of this paper is to present in brief one aspect of project 7- BUL/03/001. The project started in fall 2003 and was developed in conjunction with the Valetta Action Plan (http://www.itu.int/ITU-D/univ_access/program3.html). The latter was formulated at the end of the second ITU World Development Conference in 1998 and sought to promote universal access to basic telecommunications, broadcasting and Internet as tools of development of rural and/or remote areas. Project partners are Bulgarian Ministry of Transport and Communication, Bulgarian Telecommunication Company, Bulgarian Association of Telecenters, Telemedicine group at Bulgarian Academy of Sciences represented by Solar-Terrestrial Influences Laboratory and ITU. Project objectives are two folded: (1) in the area of telecommunications to develop, test and evaluate the effectiveness of a local, packet-based wireless access infrastructure in semi-mountainous rural area and (2) thus to provide a platform for the wide introduction of multimedia services such as telemedicine, teleeducation, etc. Telecardiology is one of project's multimedia applications.

The reasons to direct attention to development of telecardiology in rural areas are:

(a) More that half of Bulgarians live in rural areas or remote villages. They are in unfavourable conditions when accesses to IP-based technologies are considered.

(b) Cardiovascular diseases were and still are leading cause of dead for all age groups 40 and above in Bulgaria.

The main challenge of telecardiology application in this project is to develop a user friendly telecardiology environment for general practitioners (GPs). The decision to concentrate efforts on GPs was based on careful study of ecology of medical care in the country. Put in another words, on an analyses where do people look for medical help. Despite of the predictions and expectations for seeking care at tertiary level facilities at first place, the dominant numbers revealed that at first place are the visits of primary care levels (GPs). So, if we want to affect outcomes, and we really want to, our strategies should be concerned with where most people are served by the health care system, where there is the greatest potential for contributing to alleviating the burden of disease and human suffering. Understanding and taking into account the ecology of healthcare, pre-defined the choice of primary care level, i.e. GP.

2. Materials and Methods

Target region is Septemvri community with about 30 000 inhabitants, 2 towns and 12 villages most with 1000 – 2500 residents. The area is 349 km^2 including north parts of Rodopi mountains and west parts of Sredna gora mountain. Septemvri community is an ideal representative of rural area with its scarcity of public facilities and technical personal, difficult topographical and climatic conditions that make critical demands on equipment plus low level of economic activity based mainly on agriculture, high percentage of unemployment (>33%), and high calling rates per ordinary telephone line. This is a perfect place to develop and test wireless infrastructures and its multimedia applications. In addition, the floats from the spring and summer of 2005 heavily affected the region, revealing once again the necessity for wider application of state-of-the-art technologies in remote areas to secure citizens wellbeing. One more reason to choose Septemvri community was that there is no licensed cardiologist in this region. Cardiologist is visiting the region once a week for 4 hours. Thus, in order to receive an expert opinion, patients has either (a) to wait (sometimes weeks) or (b) to travel minimum 60 or even 100 kilometres to another region. At first glance the second option may be preferable, but let's not forget that most of patient with cardiovascular problems are chronics, unemployed or relatively old and for them such travel is enormous obstacle. In addition, the region is semi-mountainous, which makes travels during autumn, winter and spring rather difficult.

What has been done so far? The building of telecommunication infrastructure is at its end. It connects in a network local telecenters, GP offices, local police stations of two towns and 7 largest villages in the community, the regional Medical Center and regional Emergency Care Center in town Septemvri. In addition, the network is connected to a specialized tele-server at STIL-BAS, Bulgarian Academy of Sciences, Sofia. The network is based on wireless IP technology, normal PCs and electronic devices using TCP/IP. Frequency band of the wireless communications is 2.4 GHz. The wireless system interconnects also with public switched telephone network. The network operates at two levels providing (1) administrative and public communication service and (2) telemedicine /e-health service with a special emphasis on telecardiology and telepsychology.

The examination of pulse, blood pressure and electrocardiogram are the first and that's why the most often used tools providing clues to cardiovascular problems. Physician can easily detect many heart conditions before symptoms become apparent by measuring pulse, blood pressure and by using an electrocardiogram. That is why the precise monitoring of these parameters is essential for revealing first symptoms of coming myocardial infarct or other cardiovascular complications. In order to realize the telecardiological part of the project, GPs are supplied with portable blood pressure meters (holters) and portable 4 channel electrocardiographs (ECG holters).
Blood pressure holters are BOSO TM-2430 PC (Fig. 1).

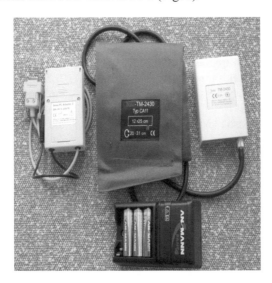

Figure 1 Blood pressure holter BOSO TM 2430

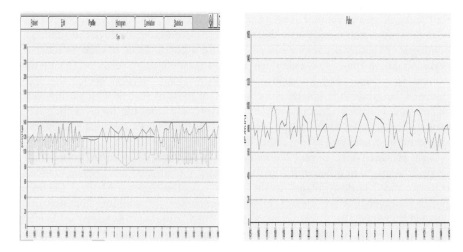

Fig. 2 Record of 24 hours blood pressure variations   **Fig. 3** Record of 24 hours pulse variations

The device measures blood pressure using oscillometric principle. It is fully automatic. Pressure measurements range from 60 to 290 mmHg for the systolic; and from 30 up to 195 mmHg for diastolic blood pressure. Possible pulse frequency range is from 20 up to 240 beats per minute. Static pressure range varies from 0 up to 300 mmHg, measurement intervals are between 1 and 30 readings per hour. The memory capacity is over 200 readings. The device is battery operated. Its weight, batteries included, is 250 g. The software is user-friendly, despite of the fact that titles that appear on the screen are in English. To make the application even easier, all titles and instructions visualized on the screen are in the process of translation in Bulgarian. The software allows saving patients' data and visualize and/or print results both in tabular or graphical format. Only a click is necessary to change the format of data presentation. Fig. 2 and 3 illustrate graphical representation of blood pressure variation and pulse during 24 hours monitoring, while figure 4 illustrate summary of the same date as a table.

The ECG holter is product of SIGNACOR Ltd, Bulgaria (Fig. 5). It is fully automatic, has 4 MB flash memory, where up to 27 hours ECG records of 4 independent channels may be saved. The holter has a sampling rate 200 s/sec, 50 Hz reject digital filter and weights less than 250 g with batteries and patient cable. Unavoidable self-diagnostic tests for (a) batteries' power and (b) electrodes' impedance, before starting the record, in order to check the electrode placement quality and an auto-calibration possibility are additional bonuses and are part of standard monitoring procedure. An extra benefit is that the software not only user-friendly but is in Bulgarian. This makes the application of the device easier and helps GPs to overcome the psychological barrier of using new, non-standard equipment.

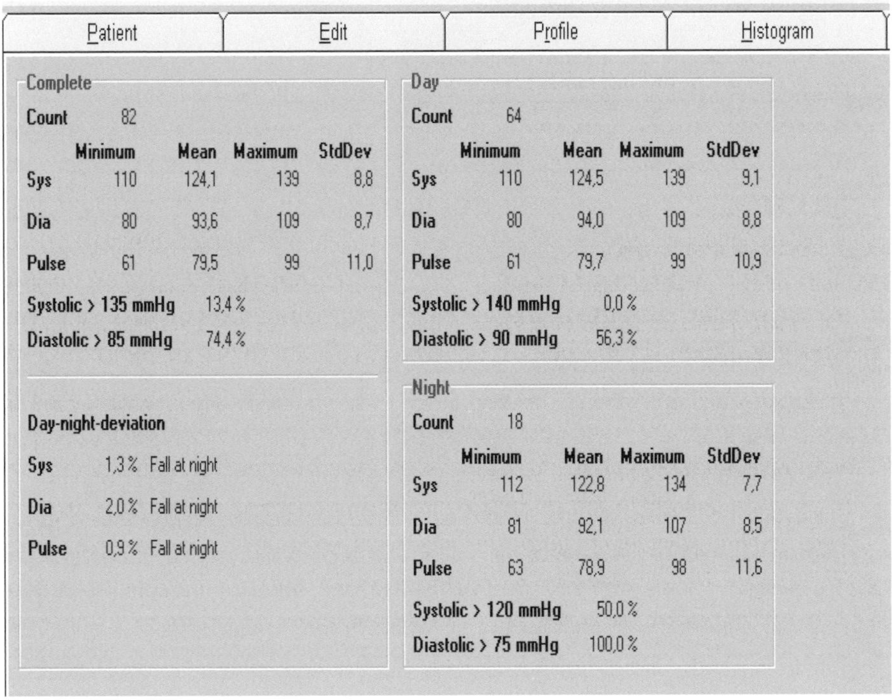

Patient	Edit	Profile	Histogram

Complete

Count 82

	Minimum	Mean	Maximum	StdDev
Sys	110	124,1	139	8,8
Dia	80	93,6	109	8,7
Pulse	61	79,5	99	11,0

Systolic > 135 mmHg   13,4 %

Diastolic > 85 mmHg   74,4 %

Day-night-deviation

Sys	1,3 % Fall at night
Dia	2,0 % Fall at night
Pulse	0,9 % Fall at night

Day

Count 64

	Minimum	Mean	Maximum	StdDev
Sys	110	124,5	139	9,1
Dia	80	94,0	109	8,8
Pulse	61	79,7	99	10,9

Systolic > 140 mmHg   0,0 %

Diastolic > 90 mmHg   56,3 %

Night

Count 18

	Minimum	Mean	Maximum	StdDev
Sys	112	122,8	134	7,7
Dia	81	92,1	107	8,5
Pulse	63	78,9	98	11,6

Systolic > 120 mmHg   50,0 %

Diastolic > 75 mmHg   100,0 %

Fig. 4. 24 hours blood pressure and pulse variations – summary table

The software allows: continuous real-time analyzes of rhythm and morphological changes in all available independent ECG leads; ST measurements; 12 Standard ECG leads reconstruction from the available channel episodes; automatic marking each time when the ECG differs from the patient's typical ECG; computing every minute averaged heart rate, RR-irregularity, QRS-width and ST deviations; automatic storage of all computed data; statistics of abnormal QRS complexes; measurements of heart rate variability; on-line monitoring on the screen at any time during the recording session; built-in editor to enter remarks and final conclusions; possibility to mark certain ECG episodes and save them as a compressed file, containing not only the marked episodes but all text and statistical data; possibility to display and print any ECG episode; generation of summary reports, histograms, tables that may be printed. Fig. 6 and 7 illustrate ECG records and marked episodes, while figures 8 and 9 - one of the patients at the beginning of 24 hours monitoring.

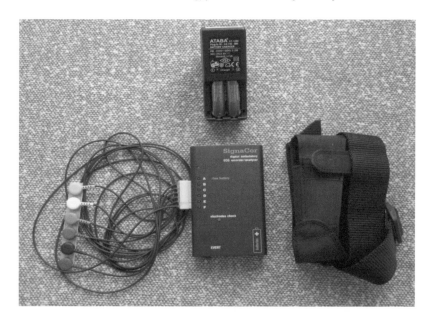

Fig. 5. ECG holter SignaCor

Using available devices, local GPs may monitor and analyze cardiovascular data and control the prescribed medication. When local GP is not skilled enough or feels necessity to consult cardiologist, he/she has the chance via his own computer or via local telecenter (if any technical support is necessary as GP offices and local telecenters are in one and the same building) to transfer abnormal parts of ECG to Septemvri Medical Centre. The feedback helps proper and fast treatment and follow-up of patients. The inclusion of this center in the net is significant achievement as this is the place where once a week the cardiologist delivers consultations. What is more, she is obliged to do these kinds of consultations. Thus local medical personnel, licensed cardiologist and patients are included in the process of tele-consultations, tele-diagnostics and tele-treatment. If and when necessary, available information may be transferred to local Emergency Medical Center, too. One additional benefit of the ECG holter software is the fact the ECG may be saved as a picture file and transfer for consultations to cardiologist who do not have the software.

It is a decision of local medical staff to whom from all patients to offer the possibility for long term monitoring and further tele-consultations.

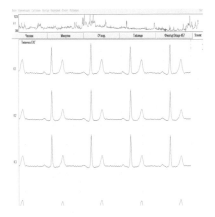

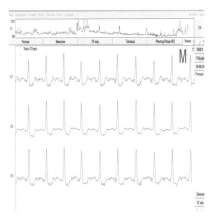

Fig. 6 ECG records   **Fig. 7** ECG records with marked abnormalities

3. Results

The telecommunication network is ready. Local telecenters and GPs offices have been equipped. GPs lacking computer skills were trained in basic computer abilities. At present they undergo training for using electronic mails, IP telephones and video connections.

After revealing the low level of computer skills of local GPs we gave up the idea to organize group training courses for the proper usage of blood pressure and ECG holter and start individual training of both GPs and nurses, if there are any in some of the villages. Individual trainings were combined with practical demonstrations. There was at least one day training for each of the devices. At the end of each training day GPs were forced to perform all steps of monitoring procedures. Figures 10 - 12 illustrate some of training sessions in Emergency Medical Center, Septemvri Medical Center and village Vetren.

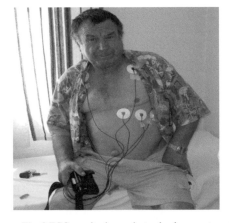

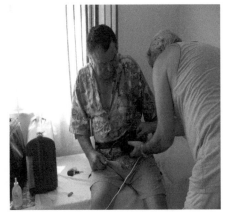

Fig. 8 ECG monitoring – electrode placement   **Fig. 9** ECG monitoring – patient ready to leave GP office

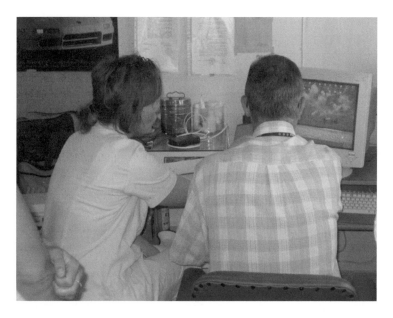

Fig. 10 Training of medical personal at regional Emergency Care Center

Realistic in our expectations, we were prepared to face significant problems during the realization of tele-cardiology applications.

Some of the problems so far are:

- Personal negative attitude or at least suspicion towards telemedicine /e-health applications and especially to distant consultations / treatment as compared to face-to-face service. This has nothing to do with GPs age, irrespective of our preliminary expectations that those GPs that are 45 yrs old and above will be more rigid in accepting new technology.
- Lack of technical experience of both medical staff and patients causes serious problems both in usage of devices and data collection, analyzes and transfer of records for consultations. Despite of the fact that most of GPs have experience with standard electrocardiographs the use of PC connected devices turned out to be a serious problem. Starting the holters, filling up patients' personal data and medical history and especially downloading results is a serious emotional obstacle for many GPs. This is one serious challenge to be overcome within next months.
- Ethical and financial problems.
- In addition, during virtual consultations people lack the nonverbal communication channel to which they are so accustomed in face-to-face communication. This is partially overcome by application of IP telephones and video connections. Thus in the process of teleconsultations, if and when necessary, colleagues communicate via IP telephones or video channels.

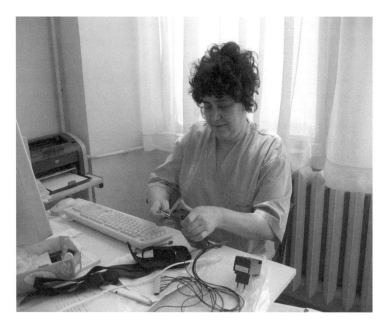

Fig. 11 Training of medical personal at regional Medical Center

The above mentioned problems forced us to re-arrange the time scheme of the project, to extend the preliminary phase and prolong project duration. Nevertheless partners believe that final outcomes will compensate all difficulties as groups that will benefit from telecardiology application are not only chronic cardiovascular patients but also patients on medications, which may affect the heart, pregnant women, patients suffering from kidney diseases, pulmonary hypertension, anorexia nervosa, narcolepsy and elderly. The latter group is especially important as congestive heart failure, is the single most frequent cause of hospitalization for people aged 65 years or older and because the percentage of elderly in our population is rapidly increasing.

As mentioned earlier the network includes one more tele-server at STIL-BAS that has to be under the supervision of Telemedicine Group and have to serve as methodological supervisor to both local GPs and Septemvri Medical Centre staff in the process of development and deployment of all telemedicine activities, i.e. from correct use of tele-cardiology equipment to precise application of software and data storage and correct fill in of electronic patient databases. Telemedicine group has also the following tasks:

(1) To study and analyze medical effect of tele-cardiology service in terms of time of treatment, time for receiving consultations, etc;

(2) To try and estimate the financial effect of telecardiology applications compared to normal face-to-face visits (reduction of health care costs by reducing the number of visits that medical staff needs to make to their patients; by cutting down on patients' journeys to health centres or specialists consultations; by reducing the length of stay in hospitals and etc.);

(3) To assess the psychological effect of telecardiology, i.e. to rate the satisfaction of the medical staff applying tele-consultations, analyzing tele-healthcare acceptance from the point of view of patients and relatives, etc.

The above mentioned analyses will be made probably at the end of 2006 when big database will be collected.

STIL-BAS tele-server may also be used for tele-education and tele-training of medical doctors and nurses from the rural area, to organize tele-conferences, tele-trading for telemedicine products, etc., as well as for organization, if and when necessary, consultations with highly qualified medical specialist in Sofia. All this is in the plans for the next year.

Having in mind the problems faced so far and fears of local GPs, since beginning of October 2005, the server will be used at first place to ensure psychological support to local GPs and medical staff as well as to organize and offer virtual psychology counselling to patients. Highly qualified specialist from Institute of Psychology at Bulgarian Academy of Sciences, the largest psychological unit in the country, are responsible for these tele-psychology supports and consultations.

4. Conclusion

This project is the first attempt to apply telecardiology services in rural area. The expected outcomes are:

- Cheap e-health service suitable to improve the quality of health care and health monitoring of patients due to faster diagnosis and treatment, reduced delay in giving medicines and performing scheduled actions, avoidance of inconvenience of travelling, highly qualified distant consultations, reduction of length of stay in hospitals, psychological comfort, etc;
- Development of advanced interactive environment for medical staff due to improved consultation and follow-up, more time available to devote to patients, reduction of waiting lists, travels and lost of time, reduction of stress and time pressure, etc;
- New knowledge concerning the acceptance of intelligent environment by patients and the influence of e-health service on life satisfaction and on satisfaction from virtual health supervision;
- Significant reduction of the part of health care budgets dedicated to home health visits.

Through this project we hope to illuminate the potential for virtual healthcare work, and to share our evolving understanding of what is truly possible, despite the prevalent myths and realities which shape our thinking about virtual diagnostics, consultations and therapy.

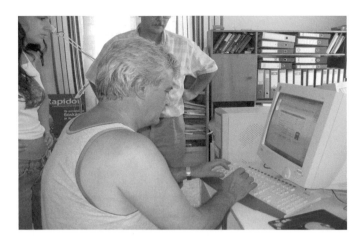

Fig. 12 Training of GP in village Vetren

Advanced Technology: Research, Application and Integration of 3D Structural Information with Multimedia Contents for Tele-virtual Dg./Therapy: Possible Use in the NATO Environment

Ivica KLAPAN [a,b,c], Ljubimko ŠIMIČIĆ [c], Sven LONČARIĆ [d,e], Mario KOVAČ [d], Ante-Zvonimir GOLEM [b,c,f], Juraj LUKINOVIĆ [a,b,c]

[a]*University Department of ENT, Head & Neck Surgery, Division of Plastic and Reconstructive Head & Neck Surgery and Rhinosinusology, Zagreb University School of Medicine, Salata 4, Zagreb, Croatia*
[b]*Zagreb University Hospital Center, Zagreb, Croatia*
[c]*Reference Center for Computer Aided Surgery and Telesurgery, Ministry of Health, Republic of Croatia, Zagreb, Croatia*
[d]*Faculty of Electrical Engineering and Computing, University of Zagreb, Croatia*
[e]*Department of Electrical and Computer Engineering, New Jersey Institute of Technology, Newark, USA*
[f]*Ministry of Health and Social Welfare Republic of Croatia*

Keywords. Computer assisted surgery, Telesurgery, Three-dimensional visualization, Endoscopy, Telemedicine, Virtual reality, Virtual endoscopy.

This work was in part supported by an unrestricted grant by the Ministry of Science and Technology, Republic of Croatia, No. 5-01-543/03-05 (Dr. Klapan)

The paper was presented at the Advanced Research Workshop «Remote Cardiology Consultations Using Advanced Medical Technology – Applications for NATO Operations», held in Zagreb, Croatia 13-16 September 2005

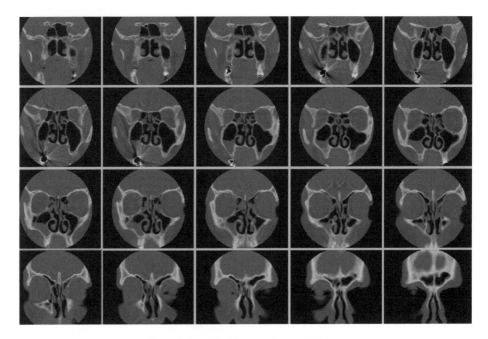

Figure 1. CT of the Nose and Paranasal Sinuses

1. Introduction

In human medicine, extremely valuable information on anatomic relationships in particular regions while planning and performing modern approaches in the surgery, such as endoscopic surgery, is provided by high quality CT or MRI diagnosis [1](Fig.1), thus contributing greatly to the safety of this kind of surgery [2].

Research in the area of 3-D image analysis, visualization, tissue modelling, and human-machine interfaces provides scientific expertise necessary for developing successful 3D-CAS (computer assisted surgery) [3], Tele-3D-CAS, and VR (virtual reality) [4,5] applications. Mentioned technologies represent a basis for realistic simulations that are useful in many areas of human activity (including medicine), and can create an impression of immersion of a physician in a non-existing, virtual environment. Such an impression of immersion can be realized in any medical institution using advanced computers and computer networks that are required for interaction between a person and a remote environment, with the goal of realizing tele-presence.

To understand the idea of 3D-CAS/VR it is necessary to recognize that the perception of surrounding world created in our brain is based on information coming from the human senses and with the help of a knowledge that is stored in our brain. The usual definition says that the impression of being present in a virtual environment (VE), such as virtual endoscopy (VE) of the patient's head, that does not exist in reality is called VR. The user/physician, has impression of presence in the virtual world and can navigate through it and manipulate virtual objects. A 3D-CAS/VR system may be designed in such a way that the user/physician, is completely immersed in the VE.

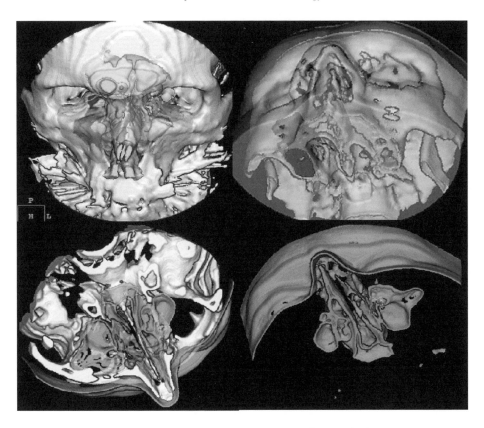

Figure 2. Our 3D models of the human head in different projections.

2. Preoperative Preparation

Use of the latest program systems enables development of 3D spatial models, exploration in various projections, simultaneous presentation of multiple model sections and, most important, model development according to open computer standards (Open Inventor). Such a preoperative preparation can be applied in a variety of program systems that can be transmitted to distant collaborating radiologic and surgical work sites for preoperative consultation as well as during the operative procedure in real time[6] (telesurgery) (Fig. 2). The real-time requirement means that the simulation must be able to follow the actions of the user that may be moving in the virtual environment. The computer system must also store in its memory a 3-D model of the virtual environment (3D-CAS models). In that case a real-time VR system will update the 3-D graphical visualization as the user moves, so that up-to-date visualization is always shown on the computer screen. For realistic simulations it is necessary for the computer to generate at least 30 such images per second, which imposes strong requirements to computer processing power.

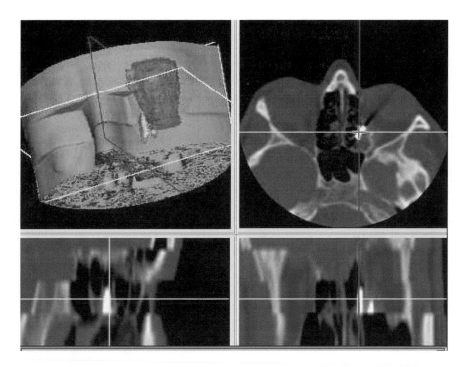

Figure 3. An example of 3D computer-assisted surgery (3D-CAS) with simulation and planning of the course of subsequent endoscopic operation (VE)

Modern technologies of exploring 3D spatial models allow for simulation of CAS / endoscopic surgery and planning the course of the future procedure (VE) or elesurgery (Tele-Virtual Endoscopy). By entering the models and navigating through the operable regions the surgeon becomes aware of the problems he will encounter during the real operation. In this way, preparation for the operation could be done including identification of the shortest and safest mode for the real operation to perform [6,7] (Fig. 3)

During the course of our Three-Dimensional Computer Assisted Functional Endoscopic Sinus Surgery (3D-C-FESS) method development, a variety of program systems were employed to design an operative field model by use of spatial volume rendering techniques (www.mef.hr/3D-CFESS). Initially, the modeling was done by use of the VolVis, Volpack/Vprender, GL Ware programs on a DEC Station 3100 computer. With the advent of 3D Viewnix V1.0 software, we started using this program, and then 3D Viewnix V1.1 system, AnalyzeAVW system, T-Vox system and OmniPro 2 system on Silicon Graphics O2, Origin200 and Origin2000 computers (Fig. 4).

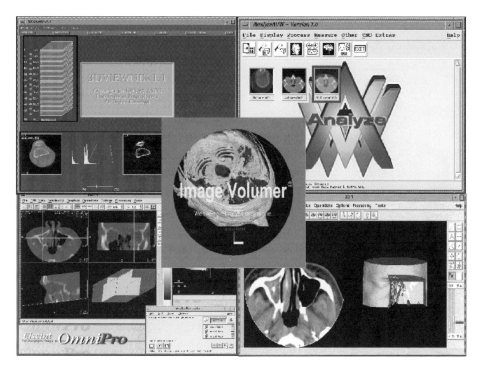

Figure 4. 3D Viewnix V1.0 and AnalyzeAVW (OmniPro 2 is shown in Fig 3)

3. Computer Assisted Diagnosis and Surgery

3D-CAS systems may be used to aid delivery of surgical procedures. In fact, the most useful systems are augmented reality systems, which combine a patient image with images obtained using various medical imaging modalities such as CT, MR, and ultrasound. Such systems for surgical delivery are used for neurosurgery, knee surgery, endoscopic ENT surgery, and breast biopsy. During mentioned procedure, the surgeon can operate the computer system by his voice (Voice Navigation). Model movements on the monitor, various projections and sections can be obtained by simple and short voice instructions during the surgery.

The system fuses computer-generated images with endoscopic image in real time. Surgical instruments have 3-D tracking sensors and the instrument position is superimposed on the video image and CT image of the patient head. The system provides guidance according to the surgically planned trajectory. The advantages of the system include reduced time for procedure, reduced training time, greater accuracy, and reduced trauma for the patient. On initial computer aided operative procedures, spatial orientation within the operative field of a 3D computer model and transfer of the particular point to the real operative field of the patient were performed by arbitrary approximation of the known reference points of the operative field anatomy [8]. In this way, the given entities were recognized on the model and in the real operative field [9]. The use of 3D spatial model of the operative field during the surgery has pointed to the

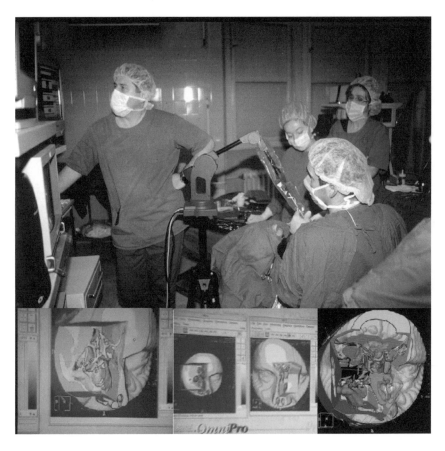

Figure 5. An example of our 3D computer assisted surgery. Advantages of VE and/or tele-VE are that there are no restrictions on the movement of virtual endoscope (it can be moved anywhere through the body), it avoids insertion of an instrument into a natural body opening or minimally invasive opening, and requires no hospitalization.

need of positioning the tip of the instrument (endoscope, forceps, etc.) within the computer model. The major problem is transmission of the real patient operative field co-ordinate system to the co-ordinate system of the computer 3D spatial model of the same patient, which has been previously designed from a series of CT images during preoperative preparation [10]. (Fig. 5).

Using a special digitalizer model and computer model, the preoperative preparation and simulation of the entire procedure can be done on the computer model of the real patient. Employing 3D digitalizer on the real procedure, the tip of the instrument (simulated endoscope) can be precisely identified in the real operative field and visualized on the computer model [5,11]. The freedom of endoscope manipulation during the procedure is not reduced because the connection is realized at the sites of instrument handle and endocamera link.

4. Computer Assisted Telesurgery

Telemedicine attempts to break the distance barrier between the provider and the patient in health-care delivery. VR is able to simulate remote environments and can therefore be applied to telemedicine. Physicians can have VR produced copy of a remote environment including the patient at their physical location. One of the simplest telemedical applications is medical teleconsultation, where physicians exchange medical information, over computer networks, with other physicians in the form of image, video, audio, and text. Teleconsultations can be used in radiology, pathology, surgery, and other medical areas. One of the most interesting telemedical applications is tele-surgery. Telesurgery is a telepresence application in medicine where the surgeon and the patient are at different locations, but such systems are still in an early research phase. Patients, who are too ill or injured to be transported to a hospital, may be operated remotely. In all these cases, there is a need for a surgeon specialist who is located at some distance.

The purpose of a tele-presence system is to create a sense of physical presence at a remote location. Tele-presence is achieved by generating sensory stimulus so that the operator has an illusion of being present at a location distant from the location of physical presence. A tele-presence system extends operator's sensory-motor facilities and problem solving abilities to a remote environment. A tele-operation system enables operation at a distant remote site by providing the local operator with necessary sensory information to simulate operator's presence at the remote location. Tele-operation is a special case of tele-presence where in addition to illusion of presence at a remote location operator also has the ability to perform certain actions or manipulations at the remote site. In this way it is possible to perform various actions in distance locations, where it is not possible to go due to a danger, prohibitive price, or a large distance. Realization of VR systems requires software (design of VE) for running VR applications in real-time. Simulations in real-time require powerful computers that can perform real-time computations required for generation of visual displays. Computer technologies allow for computer assisted surgery to be performed at distance. The basic form of telesurgery can be realized by using audio and video consultations during the procedure.

Modern equipment, such as the endo-micro cameras, show the operative field on the monitor mounted in the operating theater, however, the image can also be transmitted to a remote location by use of video transmission. The latest computer technology enables receipt of CT images from a remote location, examination of these images, development of 3D spatial models, and transfer of thus created models back to the remote location [12]. All these can be done nearly within real time. These procedures also imply preoperative consultation. During the surgery, those in the operating theater and remote consultants follow on the patient computer model the procedure images, the «live» video image generated by the endoscopic camera, and instrument movements made by the remote surgeon[6]. Simultaneous movement of the 3D spatial model on the computers connected to the system providing consultation is enabled [6,12]. It should be noted that in most cases, intraoperative consultation can be realized from two or more locations, thus utmost care should be exercised to establish proper network among them. The extreme usage of computer networks and telesurgery

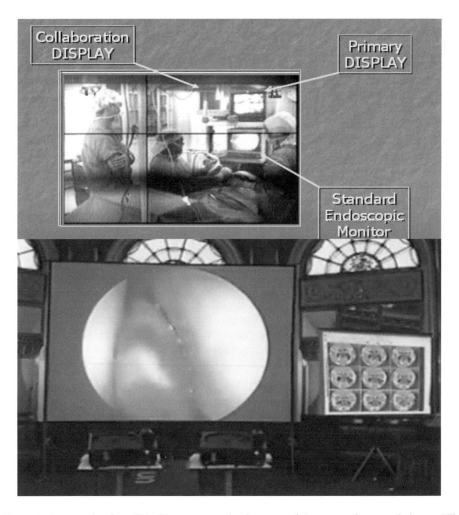

Figure 6. An example of our Tele-3D-computer assisted surgery of the nose and paranasal sinuses. VE procedure has several steps, such as: 3-D imaging of the organ of interest (e.g using CT, or MRI), 3-D preprocessing of the acquired image data (interpolation, registration), 3-D image analysis to create the model of the desired anatomical structures (segmentation), computation of the 3-D camera-target path for automatic fly-through or manual path selection, and rendering of multiple views along the computed path to create the animation (either surface or volume rendering).

implies the use of robot technologies operated by remote control. In such a way, complicated operative procedures could be carried out from distant locations. The main idea considering the use of computer networks in medicine is: *IT IS PREFERABLE TO MOVE THE DATA RATHER THAN THE PATIENT* (Fig. 6). In the future, we can expect more applications of VR in medicine. Advances in computer science will make possible more realistic simulations. VR, 3D-CAS, and Tele-3D-CAS systems of the future will find many applications in both medical diagnostics and computer-aided intervention.

5. Postoperative Analysis

3D-CAS/VR has many applications in computer-aided surgery. The four main application areas are a) surgical training and rehearsal (for education of surgeons, for rehearsal of complex surgical procedures), b) surgical planning, c) surgical rehearsal, and surgical delivery.

Surgical workstation that includes 3-D vision, dexterous precision surgical instrument manipulation, and input of force feedback sensory information. The surgeon operates in a virtual world. The use of computer technology during preoperative preparation and surgery performance allows for all relevant patient data to store during the treatment. CT images, results of other tests and examinations, computer images, 3D spatial models, and both computer and video records of the course of operation and teleoperation are stored in the computer and in CD-R devices for subsequent analysis [7] (www.mef.hr/MODERNRHINOLOGY). Also, these are highly useful in education on and practice of different approaches in surgery for surgery residents as well as for specialists in various surgical subspecialties.

The real surgery and telesurgery procedures can be subsequently analyzed and possible shortcomings defined in order to further improve operative treatment. The use of latest computer technologies enables connection between the computer 3D spatial model of the surgical field and video recording of the course of surgery to observe all critical points during the procedure, with the ultimate goal to improve future procedures and to develop such an expert system that will enable computer assisted surgery and telesurgery with due account of all the experience acquired on previous procedures. Also, using the computer recorded co-ordinate shifts of 3D digitalizer during the telesurgery procedure, an animated image of the course of surgery can be created in the form of navigation, i.e. the real patient operative field fly-through, as it was done from the very begining (from 1998) in our telesurgeries [13].

6. Computer Networks

The network is the basis for teleoperation. Very important factor for realization of 3D-CAS/Tele-3D-CAS/VR systems is a fast computer network. Fast computer networks are also the basis for telemedical applications, which may also be viewed as a kind of teleoperation systems.

7. System Implementation

In 1992, a scientific research rhinosurgical team was organized at the University Department of ENT, Head & Neck Surgery, Zagreb University School of Medicine and Zagreb University Hospital Center in Zagreb, who have developed the idea of a novel approach in head surgery. This computer aided functional endoscopic sinus microsurgery has been named 3D-C-FESS. The first 3D-C-FESS operation in Croatia was carried out at the Šalata University Department of ENT, Head & Neck Surgery in

May 1994, when a 12-year-old child, was inflicted a gunshot wound in the region of the left eye. The child was blinded on the injured eye. Six years after the 3D C-FESS surgery, the status of the left eye was completely normal, as well as the vision, which was normal bilaterally.

With due understanding and support from the University Department of ENT, Head & Neck Surgery, Zagreb University Hospital Center; Merkur University Hospital; T-Com Company; InfoNET; and SiliconMaster, in May 1996 the scientific research rhinosurgical team from the Šalata University Department of ENT, Head & Neck Surgery organized and successfully conducted the first distant radiologic-surgical consultation (teleradiology) within the frame of the 3D-C-FESS project. The consultation was performed before the operative procedure between two distant clinical work posts in Zagreb (Šalata University Department of ENT, Head & Neck Surgery and Merkur University Hospital) (outline/network topology).

In 1998, and on several occasions thereafter, the team conducted a number of first tele-3D-computer asssisted operations (Fig. 7) as unique procedures of the type not only in Croatia but worldwide [6,12]. (www.mef.hr/MODERNRHINOLOGY).

References

[1   Mladina R, Hat J, Klapan I, Heinzel B. An endoscopic approach to metallic foreign bodies of the nose and paranasal sinuses. Am J Otolaryngol, 1995, 16(4):276-279.

[2] Rišavi R, Klapan I, Handžić-Ćuk J, Barčan T. Our experience with FESS in children. Int J Pediatric Otolaryngol, 1998, 43:271-275.

[3] Elolf E, Tatagiba M, Samii M. 3D-computer tomographic reconstruction: planning tool for surgery of skull base pathologies. Comput Aided Surg,1998, 3:89-94.

[4] Holtel MR, Burgess LP, Jones SB. Virtual reality and technologic solutions in otolaryngology. Otolaryngol Head Neck Surg, 1999, 121:181.

[5] Klapan I, Šimičić Lj, Rišavi R, Bešenski N, Bumber Ž, Stiglmajer N, Janjanin S. Dynamic 3D computer-assisted reconstruction of metallic retrobulbar foreign body for diagnostic and surgical purposes. Case report: orbital injury with ethmoid bone involvement. Orbit, 2001, 20:35-49.

[6] Klapan I, Šimičić Lj, Rišavi R, Pasari K, Sruk V, Schwarz D, Barišić J. Real time transfer of live video images in parallel with three-dimensional modeling of the surgical field in computer-assisted telesurgery. J Telemed Telecare, 2002,8 :125-130.

[7] Klapan I, Šimičić Lj, Bešenski N Bumber Ž, Janjanin S, Rišavi R, Mladina R. Application of 3D-computer assisted techniques to sinonasal pathology. Case report: war wounds of paranasal sinuses with metallic foreign bodies. Am J Otolaryngol, 2002, 23:27-34.

[8] Klimek L, Mosges M, Schlondorff G, Mann W. Development of computer-aided surgery for otorhinolaryngology. Comput Aided Surg, 1998, 3:194-201.

[9] Mann W, Klimek L. Indications for computer-assisted surgery in otorhinolaryngology. Comput Aided Surg 3,1998, 202-204.

[10] Anon J. Computer-aided endoscopic sinus surgery. Laryngoscope 108:949-961, 1998.

[11] Olson G, Citardi M. Image-guided functional endoscopic sinus surgery. Otolaryngol Head Neck Surg, 1999, 121:187.

[12] Klapan I, Šimičić Lj, Rišavi R, Bešenski N, Pasarić K, Gortan D, Janjanin S, Pavić D, Vranješ Ž. Tele-3D computer assisted functional endoscopic sinus surgery: new dimension in the surgery of the nose and paranasal sinuses. Otolaryngol Head Neck Surg, 2002, 127:549-557.

[13] Klapan I, Vranješ Ž, Rišavi R, Šimičić Lj. Computer assisted surgery and telesurgery in otorhinolaryngology. Telemedicine (ed. Klapan I, Čikeš I), Telemedicine Association Zagreb, 2005.

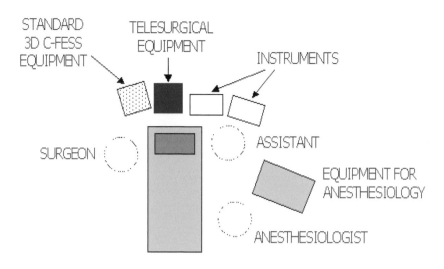

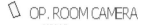

Figure 7. An example of our Tele-3D-C-FESS surgery initially performed in 1998

Remote Cardiology Consultations Using Advanced Medical Technology
I. Klapan and R. Poropatich (Eds.)
IOS Press, 2006

ICT in Telemedicine/Telecardiology System on Croatian Islands: the Potential Utility of This Technology on a Regional Basis in the South-eastern Europe

Mario KOVAČ [a], Ivica KLAPAN [b,c,d]

[a] Faculty of Electrical Engineering and Computing, University of Zagreb, Croatia
[b] University Department of ENT, Head & Neck Surgery, Division of Plastic and Reconstructive Head & Neck Surgery and Rhinosinusology, Salata 4, Zagreb University School of Medicine
[c] Zagreb University Hospital Center, Zagreb, Croatia
[d] Reference Center for Computer Aided Surgery and Telesurgery, Ministry of Health, Salata 4, Zagreb, Croatia

Keywords. Telemedicine, Computer System, Business Organization, Image Analysis, Security

The paper was presented at the Advanced Research Workshop «Remote Cardiology Consultations Using Advanced Medical Technology – Applications for NATO Operations», held in Zagreb, Croatia 13-16 September 2005

1. Introduction

Ministry of Health, Republic of Croatia has recently introduced a brand new telemedicine/telecardiology system. This system (referred to as telemed system in further text) is primarily focused to cover medical needs of patients residing on or visiting croatian islands. Implementation of the system is currently in phase one, where all medical, legal, organizational and technical aspects of the system will be analyzed. It does not have to be mentioned that each and every aspect of the system is complex and important and detailed analysis requires large amount of time and resources. In this work we present only one aspect of the system: organization of the system and potential to use this system in a region.

System organization is flexible and independant, can operate stand-alone or linked to some other medical system. This results in several exciting options for expansion. First and most obvious option is that the system is replicated in other application area (e.g. military remote medical centers, mountain areas, etc). Second option is that the system is merged with other medical systems. This option is especially attractive since it can result in major operational savings due to the fact that two medical information systems share many common resources and services. Yet another option is to allow sharing of experts with other telemed systems allowing consultations and experts outsourcing. This options is also attractive for several SE European regions.

From the above it is clear that telemed system that is being built for Croatian islands can be viewed as attractive medical system for use in other regions in SE Europe.

2. System Architecture

The system we are describing is designed as multi-star like network. In the centers of each star there is a strong medical center with experts in various medical areas. Links from those centers go to remote locations where patients are treated. Centers itsef are inter-connected allowing sharing of resources and intelligent time management. Interconnection of expert centers also serves for redundancy purposes in case one of the centers is not capable of delivering required medical help for whatever reason.

In Figure 1. we can see this organization. It is simple, implemented using standard network access and can be mapped to almost every other region. One can notice that all nodes are virtually connected to all other nodes thus enabling multiple connections and allowing redundancy in case of problems.

The Telecommunication/telemedicine System for Support of Emergency Medical Service on Selected Croatian Islands includes installation of the communication equipment and videoconference systems (with additional equipment) at [7] locations on selected Croatian Islands, with system centers in Split [7] and Zagreb [7] (expert medical sites/university departments), and one additional research site. Split and Zagreb centers are primary expert locations that connect several institutions from University hospital center Split and University hospital center Zagreb. Out of many islands that will require such infrastructure, islands of Hvar, Brac, Korcula and Vis have been chosen for the first phase.

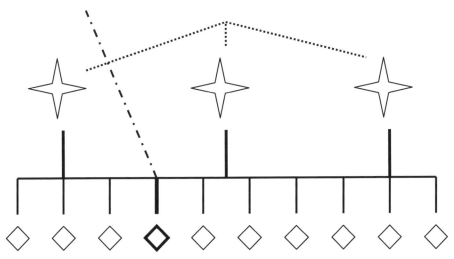

Figure 1. Network of Centers (4 point stars) and local units (diamonds)

In the same Figure we can see possible links to other medical networks painted with dotted lines. In our architecture this link can be used for several purposes.

First and most obvious purpose is link to Croatian medical information system [6,7]. As we said earlier, our system can operate standalone but it is of mutual interest that certain information in the system is synchronized with the general medical information system. When we think of minimal information that should be exchanged then we are talking about financial transactions required for system operation and passing of certain medical information about patients. Due to the fact that Croatia is currently undergoing a major change in organization of medical information system infrastructure this link will bring many benefits to the system itself. This link will be custom built and tailored to needs of Croatian medical information system. We however are already preparing the same for other users of this telemed system. In our approach we can custom design link to any foreign medical system allowing both medical and financial control of services provided for selected groups of users.

Another purpose of those links is to enable that our medical experts can become active participants in other regional telemed networks. It has been shown in the past that Croatian medical experts are highly respected and that they are consulted quite often by their colleagues from all over the world. Providing this link allows consultations to be virtually enabled at all times.

What is also visible from the simple image in Figure 1 is that we can allow that expert help is provided from some other medical center that is not part of the Croatian network (dot-dash line). This is especially interesting when doctors have to ask for medical opinion from certain certified experts (an example would be NATO forces using local centers but requiring diagnoses to be provided by NATO certified centers, another example is in cases of emergencies or disasters where additional experts are required to cover the need in particular time frame).

By analizing the above we claim that our telemed system infrastructure, although created for civil purposes, can easily be mapped to any NATO specified architecture and/or be used as a part of any regional telemedicine network.

3. Image analysis

In order to optimize costs of running the system and reduce overall system requirements we have started the detailed analysis of medical images that are and will be used in the system. One must not foget that there are technological limitations in using the technology. Medical images are key differentiator feature between simple and advanced medical systems. Correct understanding of processes that are part of the medical system architecture, underlying algorithms and procedures are of utmost importance if one wants to introduce usage of medical imaging in healthcare system [2,4,5] Currently there are several image coding standards that are being used in medical applications. All those standards have been developed and introduced to the market by the consortium of experts from various companies under the name of JPEG (Joint Photographic Expert Group). Three standards that are being used are ISO/IEC IS 10918, ISO/IEC IS 14495 and ISO/IEC IS 15444 but usually they are referred to as JPEG, JPEG-LS and JPEG2000 respectively.

Medical images represent a small subset of all images that require some sort of compression to be efficiently used in computer systems and transmitted over the network. Certain images that are of key importance may even not be compressed to allow extraction of information and analysis at any given time in the future. Due to the imperfection of human visual system in many cases one can compress image and significantly reduce it's size while still preserving quality required for proper medical analysis. DICOM standard is one example of complex data descriptor that is being used to exchange medical data (and images) and it allows uncompressed as well as compressed images to be used.

All image compression algorithms can be placed in two groups: lossless and lossy [3]. By definition, lossless algorithms will compress image and once the image is decompressed it will be identical to the original. The advantage of such approach is that compressed images are much smaller in size then originals. On the other side, lossy algorithms will not be able to restore the image to be identical to the original but with proper selection of parameters the image might be indistinguishably similar to the original to the normal viewer. The algorithms applied in lossy approach take the advantage of imperfection of human visual system to extract data that is not visible to the human and therefore reducing the size while preserving the quality as much as possible. One must note that deep compression (compression that results in high compression ratios) will inevitably introduce visible differences. In certain applications even this is tolerable due to the fact that only general overview of the image is required rather then detailed analysis.

The key issue that must be well defined before using processed digital images is the definition of the required quality and robustness. It is obvious that if we use only unprocessed and uncompressed images that we will have highest possible quality and robustness. Unfortunately, we cannot expect that the costs of such principle will be affordable for distributed and mass usage. For the most important images we can use lossless compression algorithms. Table 1 briefly summarizes some major benefits of different image coding algorithms that can be used in today's telemed system.

Table 1. Comparison of different image coding algorithms

	JPEG 2000	JPEG-LS	JPEG	MPEG-4 VTC	PNG
lossless compression performance	+++	++++	+	-	+++
lossy compression performance	+++++	+	+++	++++	-
progressive bitstreams	+++++	-	++	+++	+
Region of Interest (ROI) coding	+++	-	-	+	-
arbitrary shaped objects	-	-	-	++	-
random access	++	-	-	-	-
low complexity	++	+++++	+++++	+	+++
error resilience	+++	++	++	+++	+
non-iterative rate control	+++	-	-	+	-
genericity	+++	+++	++	++	+++

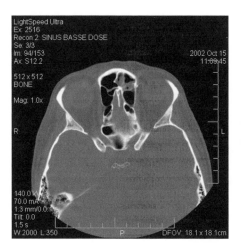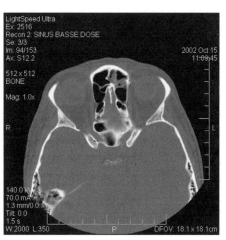

Figure 2. Comparison of original and compressed medical image (lossless compression)

What can be seen from Figure 2. is an example of lossless image compression applied to a medical image. The quality of the image is completely preserved but the size of the compressed image is few times smaller (in this example the original image on the left is 258KB while the compressed image on the right is 80KB). Thus, by using this approach communication bandwith and costs can be reduced. Larger compression ratios could be achieved using lossy coding that can be applied to images that are not highly sensitive to errors (e.g. dermatology).

In the figure (Figure 3) we demonstrate very efficient use of simple lossy compression algorithms. Top figure shows an original image taken without compression. Analysis of this type of images does not require very fine details. In the bottom left image we have applied relatively high compression (compression ratio is 57:1) and most of the information in the image is still of good quality. In the bottom right image we have used even higher compression (94:1) and even this image is good enough for certain applications. From the above we have demonstrated the efficiency of the technology that is available and that is part of our telemedicine system.

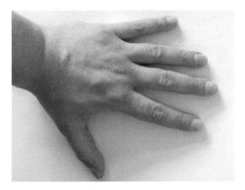

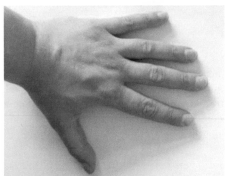 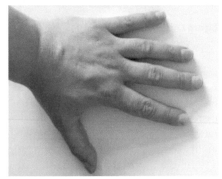

Figure 3. Comparison of compressed medical image using lossy algorithms and large compression ratios (top: uncompressed original, bottom left: compressed with ratio 57:1, bottom right: compressed with ratio 94:1)

4. Smart card privacy and security

Privacy and security of information and communication have been placed on the top of our list of system requirements [1]. In order to protect personal or classified data we have decided to organize our system to use high levels of security. As a key differentiator we have introduced smart card based system for processing of sensitive information. By introducing smart cards we can allow features such as: digital signatures and certificates, secure and encrypted message passing, logging of communication for potential legal analyis and many other.

In our system architecture we have been following major international recommendations for telemed system (such as CPME guidelines for telemedicine and others). There are many procedures in a telemed system that require identification, signatures and other types of special data handling.

5. Conclusions

The system organization is flexible and independant, can operate stand-alone or linked to some other medical system. This results in several exciting options for expansion. First option is that the system is replicated in other application area (e.g. military remote medical centers). Second option is that the system is merged with other medical systems. Another option is to allow sharing of experts with other telemed systems allowing consultations and experts outsourcing. This options is also attractive for several SE European regions. Our telemed system infrastructure, although created for civil purposes, can easily be mapped to any NATO specified architecture and/or be used as a part of any regional telemedicine network.

In order to optimize costs of running the system and reduce overall system requirements we have started the detailed analysis of medical images that are and will be used in the system. Medical images are key differentiator feature between simple and advanced medical systems. Correct understanding of processes that are part of the medical system architecture, underlying algorithms and procedures are of utmost importance if one wants to introduce usage of medical imaging in healthcare system.

Privacy and security of information and communication have been placed on the top of our list of system requirements. In order to protect personal or classified data we have decided to organize our system to use high levels of security. As a key differentiator we have introduced smart card based system for processing of sensitive information. By introducing smart cards we can allow features such as: digital signatures and certificates, secure and encrypted message passing, logging of communication for potential legal analyis and many other.

References

[1] Kalpić, Damir; Mornar, Vedran; Kovač, Mario. *Personal authentication and privacy protection on Internet,* 2nd Croatian Congress of Telemedicine with International Participation / Klapan, Ivica ; Kovač, Mario (ed.), Zagreb, 2004. 42-43

[2] Kovač, Mario. *Efficient Use of Medical Images* , 2nd Croatian Congress of Telemedicine with International Participation / Klapan, Ivica ; Kovač, Mario (ed.), Zagreb, 2004. 44-45

[3] Kovač, Mario. *Benefits of MPEG multimedia communications* , Book of Abstracts – 1st Croatian Congress of Telemedicine with International Participation / Klapan, Ivica (ed.), Makarska, 2002.

[4] Knezović, Josip; Kovač, Mario, *Gradient Based Selective Weighting of Neighboring Pixels for Predictive Lossless Image Coding* , Proceedings of the 25th International Conference on INFORMATION TECHNOLOGY INTERFACES, Cavtat, Croatia, June 16-19, 2003

[5] Kovač, Mario; Ranganathan, N. *VLSI circuit structure for implementing JPEG image compression standard*, US PATENT

[6] Kalpić, Damir; Mornar, Vedran; Kovač, Mario; Fertalj, Krešimir; Medved, Ivica; Šikić, Krešimir; Petković, Mario. *Analysis and report on purchase of integrated hospital information system of the Republic of Croatia,* Ver 3.4., 2004

[7] Kalpić, Damir; Mornar, Vedran; Kovač, Mario; Fertalj, Krešimir; Medved, Ivica; Šikić, Krešimir; Petković, Mario. *Analysis and report on implementation of primary medical care information system of the Republic of Croatia*, Ver 2.0, 2004

[8] First Croatian Congress of Telemedicine, www.mef.hr/telmed-ma2002, Makarska, 2002

[9] Second Croatian Congress of Telemedicine, www.mef.hr/telmedzg04, Zagreb, 2004.

Remote Cardiology Consultations Using Advanced Medical Technology
I. Klapan and R. Poropatich (Eds.)
IOS Press, 2006

The Future isn't What It Used to Be—
(Applying New Technologies in Health Care)

David LAM [a], Ronald POROPATICH [b]

[a] *U.S. Army Telemedicine and Advanced Technology Research Center, Ft. Detrick*
Maryland and University of Maryland School of Medicine, National Study Center for
Trauma and Emergency Medical Services, Baltimore, Maryland
[b] *U.S. Army Telemedicine and Advanced Technology Research Center, Ft. Detrick*
Maryland

Abstract. The field of advanced medical technology is rapidly changing, so much that the concept of what the future holds has changed radically in recent years. That which was seen as "cutting edge" a few years ago has now become almost routine. Some of the newer concepts currently being researched by the U.S. Army's Telemedicine and Advanced Technology Research Center (TATRC) which may prove to be the drivers for new medical applications and business practices will be discussed.

The paper was presented at the Advanced Research Workshop «Remote Cardiology Consultations Using Advanced Medical Technology – Applications for NATO Operations», held in Zagreb, Croatia 13-16 September 2005

1. Introduction

Many individuals who are currently working with the issue of applying Advanced Medical Technology to clinical practice still consider Teleconsultation or Teleradiology to be futuristic and advanced, when in fact these technologies are increasingly becoming part of routine medical care throughout the world. This paper will discuss some of the newer technologies and applications on the horizon which are being investigated by the TATRC, and which may prove to have wide applicability to the future of medical practice.

2. Discussion

It is becoming increasingly frequent in conferences and meetings such as this one to hear references to "traditional Telemedicine" or "classic Teleconsultation". For those of us who have been working to develop and install Telemedicine systems which we see as having the potential to change the way medicine is practiced, this reference is sometimes a bit jolting. However, it is true. Those programs and capabilities which we saw several years ago as being futuristic and innovative are no longer so; they have been increasingly generally adopted as a routine part of the medical armamentarium. Though they are not necessarily applied in all specialties or in all regions of the world, the technology and the business rules needed to make them effective have rapidly reached maturity. Teleconsultation, Teledermatology, Teleradiology, Telepathology, Telecardiology, and the other Tele....ologies are playing and will continue to play an increasingly important part in healthcare, but they are no longer the symbol of the most advanced medical technology available.

It is important for us and for our patients that we do not remain wedded perpetually to the past, but that we constantly seek out new and improved ways to provide the best medical care to our patients. In this paper, we intend to discuss only a few of the many projects and advanced medical technologies currently being investigated by the U.S. Army Telemedicine and Advanced Technology Research Center (TATRC), which we believe will potentially have a great impact on the future of healthcare. It is not possible in the space allotted to discuss even one project in detail, much less all of TATRC's 250+ current projects. While many of our efforts have a military orientation, we fully expect that most will eventually also have civil utilization, particularly in today's world of widespread terrorist activities, inequality of medical provider distribution, limitations on the availability of medical providers, and increasing trauma incidence. However, it is the impact of these technologies on the way medicine is practiced, rather than the technologies themselves, which is of most interest.

The technologies we wish to discuss fall into seven general technology areas:
- Medical Imaging
- Medicine Over Long Distances
- Medical Informatics
- Training and Educational Systems
- Sensors and Robotics
- Communications Infrastructure
- Operating Rooms of the Future

In the area of medical imaging, we are all familiar with CAT Scans, MRI Scans, and 3-D (and now 4-D) Ultrasound. All have contributed, and will continue to do so, to the improvement of medical diagnosis and treatment. But, once again, neither these modalities nor PET Scans are the newest technology being investigated. We are now looking intensively at the potential impact of a relatively new concept called volumetric CT, or multidetector CT. This technology is not completely new, having been available for several years, but its implications and impact have potentially significant implications for the way we practice medicine. As the number of detectors in a machine increases (64 slice scanners are increasingly in use), the potential data output is significantly improved. This technology produces resolutions 2-5 times greater than conventional CT, and may soon replace diagnostic catheterization for cardiac disease. It provides us with an opportunity to investigate new applications, including ultra-high resolution anatomical studies and dynamic imaging in vivo. Volumetric imaging has the potential to significantly change our clinical and business practices, and our patients deserve our best efforts to find out how and why this new technology should be used.

In the technology area of practicing medicine over long distances, we adddress the topic of "classical telemedicine" and ways to improve its practice. The equipment needed to carry out successful Teleconsultation continues to be reduced in size, complexity, and cost. New technology improves daily our ability to carry out the various "tele…ologies". As technological advances continue, this capability is increasingly within reach of nearly all practitioners. Unfortunately, though the technology is available and the business practices are known, actual implementation of these practices in pre-existing medical practices has proven difficult. There is an inherent bias in human society (and medicine is no exception) to continue to do things "the way we always have", and when changes are made the tendency is to simply modify the old ways of doing business rather than replacing the old ways. This is a primary reason that nearly all of our societal structures (business, social, and medical) so significantly lag the pace of technological changes which they only slowly adopt [1]. We believe that Telemedicine has the potential to allow us to practice in new ways, rather than simply to allow us to automate the old way we have always practiced. Thus, our major emphasis in this area is on improved business practices and implementation, rather than focusing solely on the technological aspects of the issue.

Medical informatics has a great potential, if used correctly, to change the way we will practice in the future. In both the military and the civil emergency setting, the care given by the first responder has been initially recorded on paper, which can easily be destroyed, lost, or damaged. To improve this situation for the military, we have developed the Battlefield Medical Information System-Tactical (BMIS-T) [2]. BMIS-T is a point-of-care hand-held Personal Digital Assistant (PDA) which enables providers to record, store, retrieve and transmit the essential elements of patient encounters. It includes reference materials, diagnostic and treatment decision aids, and logistic support software, and it facilitates patient care & skill sustainment training, BMIS-T has the flexibility to incorporate new procedures and protocols & medical databases. Currently, the device provides various databanks which can be populated before deployment, such as the immunization status and previous health status of all personnel in the unit. Work is currently ongoing to make this device usable totally hands-free. All data input to the BMIS-T can either be output to an electronic "dogtag" which travels with the patient to the next level of care, or can be input directly into the Army's central medical information system. This technology has significant potential impact on the business practices of all primary responders, both civil and military, and is in increasing widespread civilian usage.

Numerous efforts are ongoing at TATRC to produce innovative and effective training devices which can improve initial and refresher training to medical personnel at all levels of professionalism. One example is the Virgil Chest Tube Training Device. Developed by the Center for Integration of Medicine & Innovative Technology (CIMIT), of Boston, Massachusetts, this device: 1) Extends the limits of human computer interactions permitting realistic medical scenarios for safe, risk free familiarization & competency testing without the need for training on animals or humans, and; 2) Combines the use of a realistic mannequin with a PC-based graphical interface. During training, this device: tracks the internal position of chest darts and chest tubes; provides realistic force feedback during the skin incision; dissection through intercostal muscle and pleura, and subsequent placement of a chest tube; and provides instant feedback to the student as to the success or failure of his intervention. [3]

Sensors and Robotics are the focus of a large proportion of the TATRC program. In the area of robotics, our efforts range from true robotic surgery, such as that of which the Da Vinci surgical Robot is capable [4] to Robotic Evacuation Vehicles [5]. "The ultimate goal of our research program in Autonomous Combat Casualty Care is to minimize exposure of medical providers and soldier first responders to the emerging hazards of modern warfare and reduction in the medical footprint deployed to a combat zone, while continuing to provide our soldiers the best possible medical care. In the future we envision the use of robots to assist our medical personnel to locate casualties, determine their degree of injury, move them to safety, provide initial care, place them in a life-supporting "Trauma Pod" [6-8], and evacuate them to more definitive care." Once the stuff of fiction, the concept of a surgeon many miles away from a patient actually performing surgery with the use of a robot has now been demonstrated clinically. Full development of such a capability may provide a mechanism to perform life-saving surgery in hazardous situations, whether in peace or war, without hazarding the life of the surgeon, or requiring the movement of the surgeon or the patient over long distances. Thus, life-saving surgery may be made available during the "golden hour", regardless of the cause of the injury. Autonomous or semi-autonomous casualty treatment systems are currently in prototype form, and include evacuation robotic (unmanned) vehicles with physiological monitoring and telemedicine capabilities built-in to them. [9] The ability to monitor patients' physiological condition before, during, and after injury, as well as during transport will be facilitated by work being done by General Dynamics Corporation to outfit the soldier of the future with wired uniforms that monitor heart rates and respiration. Other similar ongoing work involves: "Smart Skin"/ "Smart Shirt" Technologies which will constantly monitor and forward vital signs and injury information; Intelligent Agent monitors which will work with those technologies to send data only when abnormal or when queried [10]; and a new Battle Dress Uniform with new antibacterial and hemorrhage control elements impregnated in the uniform/armor. These elements may consist of Bacteriophages, tourniquets and procoagulants (fibrin foam), among other new concepts.

One of the major problems involved in providing advanced medical care in far-off, war-torn, or disaster-stricken areas is that of providing communications means. If computer or telephone land-lines and cell phone nodes are not available today, only satellite or radio communications are viable means of providing the required bandwidth for Telemedicine support. The Helios Project [11] is investigating one way of providing viable communications for the Army in such a situation, and TATRC is looking into how it could be utilized for medical purposes. This project involves the deployment of one or more unmanned long-duration aerial platforms which can serve as mobile transmit/receive nodes, providing a rapidly deployable "Communications Backbone in the Sky" which can be used to provide Broad Band, G-3 Mobile, Narrow Band, or direct broadcast communications. These systems will enable reliable, rapidly deployable access to remote patients without a costly/lengthy network build up—they will be able to be deployed rapidly and relatively inexpensively to provide this support. If this concept is successful, it may, in conjunction with work ongoing in mobile robotic telesurgery, have great impact on civilian as well as military medicine. Quality, accessible surgical care may be made available through this mechanism to underserved rural populations, or to isolated extreme environments, not to mention in case of man-made or natural disasters. As far-fetched as this concept of an ultra-high communications tower may seem, we are living in a time where the impossible is now the probable. The aircraft is slow- flying and ultra-light. A solar array is the aircraft's primary power source, and will enable it to remain aloft during daylight hours. Long flight times will require a very lightweight energy storage system based on a fuel cell concept. The next step in development of the platform is the Helios 2 that will reach altitudes of 100 kilometers and carry a 700-pound payload.

We are also heavily involved in the development of future operating rooms, what we call Operating Rooms of the Future. We are designing new integrated OR systems which will: Improve patient safety; Emphasize minimally invasive surgery; Rely on image guided surgery; Make improved use of integrated imaging modalities; Improve efficiency; Improve training/education; and generally Improve patient outcomes. There is not available enough space in this paper to go into detail about these efforts. [12]

So what is the point of all this? Simply that all of us who are interested in patient well-being and outcome need to keep our minds open. Technology cannot and will not stand still. We cannot rest on our laurels—Telemedicine and Telecardiology are important, and will in our opinion play a great role in medical care in the future, but they are no longer cutting edge technologies. We must keep up with the new technologies being developed, evaluate them for clinical relevance and applicability, and then figure out ways to incorporate them into a better way of providing better health care. As has been stated before, we must use this advanced technology to change *how* we do things… not just to automate existing processes. We have to work smarter, not just better.

If you want to know what the future holds for medical care, read some good science fiction. We don't have Star Trek's Tricorder yet (we are working on developing its basic principles), but many of the other medical advances foreseen in science fiction of 30 years ago have come to fruition—who knows what new advances will be seen in the next two or three decades? We owe it to our patients to keep on the forefront of this development wave. Advanced Medical Technology has left the launching pad, and isn't going to stop climbing onward for many years. We need to decide if we will pilot these developments or simply go along for the ride.

References

[1]   Larry Downes, and Chunka Mui ; "Unleashing the Killer App :Digital Strategies for Market Dominance".
      On Web at: http://www.killer-apps.com/
[2]   Morris, Tommy; "BMIS-T". On Web at:
      www.projectmesa.org/ftp/SSG_SA/SA06_Ottawa_2003/ BMIST%20Handout%20April%202003.pdf
[3]   Center for Integration of Medicine & Innovative Technology (CIMIT); VIRGIL; on web at:
      http://www.medicalsim.org/virgil.htm
[4]   Intuitive Surgical Corporation; " Da Vinci, Surgical System"; on web at:
      http://www.intuitivesurgical.com/products/da_vinci.html
[5]   Gilbert, Gary, et al; "Army Medical Robotics Research"; Revue Internationale Des Services De Sante Des

Forces Armees"; 78(2):105-112.
[6]   Elias, Paul; "Pentagon Invests in Unmanned "Trauma Pod"; Associated Press 28 March 2005; On Web at:
      http://www.usatoday.com/tech/news/2005-03-28-trauma-pod-pentagon_x.htm?csp=34&POE=click-refer
[7]   UMBC Research; "UMBC Ebiquity Project: "Trauma Pod""; on Web at:
      http://ebiquity.umbc.edu/project/html/id/63/
[8]   Trauma Pod conceptual video on Web at: http://www.xvivo.net/Medical2004/Index.html
[9]   PolarTec Corporation, "Wear-and-Forget Physiological Sensing System
      for Combat Casualty Care"; on Web at: http://www.polartec.com/contentmgr/showdetails.php/id/982
[10] Brower, J. Michael, "Vitality Signs"; Military Medical Technology 8(5); 1 Aug 2004: On Web at:
      http://www.military-medical-technology. com/ article.cfm?DocID=560??
[11] Helios: On web at: http://www.aerovironment.com/area-aircraft/unmanned.html
[12] Rattner, David, and Park, Adrian; "Advanced Devices for the Operating Room of the Future"; Seminars in
      Laparoscopic Surgery; 10(2): 85-89, June 2003.

PacRim Pediatric Heartsounds Trial: Store-and-Forward Pediatric Telecardiology Evaluation with Echocardiographic Validation

MAJ C. Becket MAHNKE, LTC Michael P. MULREANY

Medical Corps, U.S. Army, Tripler Army Medical Center, Pediatric Dept.,
1 Jarrett White Rd, Honolulu, HI 96859-5000

Abstract. Background: Heart murmurs are found in more than 50% of children, yet less than 1% of children are born with congenital heart disease. The auscultation skills of the general practitioners responsible for routine child care are suboptimal, however, leading to frequent referral to pediatric cardiologists for evaluation. Pediatric cardiologists can quickly and accurately diagnose innocent murmurs with physical examination only, thereby avoiding further diagnostic testing. Patients living in remote regions without pediatric cardiology support require evacuation to medical centers, which can delay diagnosis, lead to family stress, and result in significant financial expenditure for travel. Using a digital recording stethoscope and our store-and-forward telemedicine system, we developed a pediatric telecardiology system to allow for remote cardiac auscultation. We hypothesized that such a system could accurately classify auscultatory findings as normal/innocent murmur or pathologic, thereby reducing the need for many evacuations and allowing more timely evaluation of patients with cardiac pathology.

Methods: Patients undergoing evaluation in the pediatric cardiology clinic at Tripler Army Medical Center underwent standard physical examination and complete echocardiography to establish a definitive cardiac diagnosis. Using a commercially available digital stethoscope attached to a handheld PDA, study participants also had 20-second digital heartsound recordings acquired from standard cardiac auscultation areas while both upright and supine. Heartsounds were uploaded to our store-and-forward telemedicine system, allowing for playback in a manner similar to standard clinical auscultation via a custom graphical user interface. Pediatric cardiologists, blinded to all other clinical information, evaluated each heartsound dataset and classified the case as either normal or pathologic.

Results: To date, 41 pediatric patients have been evaluated (24 with normal/innocent murmurs, 17 with cardiac pathology), each of which interpreted by 3 pediatric cardiologists (total of 123 cases). When compared to echocardiographic results, 86% (106/123) of the cases were accurately classified as either normal/innocent murmur or pathologic. Nine cases with pathology were misclassified as normal/innocent murmur (sensitivity 84%). Eight cases were classified as pathologic (specificity 88%) when the findings were normal/innocent murmur.

Conclusions: Digital heartsound recordings evaluated in our store-and-forward telecardiology system can determine normal from pathologic auscultatory findings with a high degree of accuracy. Such a system has the potential to significantly decrease travel expenditures and reduce diagnostic delays for patients requiring pediatric cardiology evaluation. Further refinements to our heartsound system are in progress and are expected to further improve the accuracy of remote cardiac auscultation.

Funding: This work was supported by the US Army Medical Research and Materiel Command under MIPR #4ETCHM4065. Opinions, interpretations, conclusions and recommendations are those of the authors and are not necessarily endorsed by the US Army.

The paper was presented at the Advanced Research Workshop «Remote Cardiology Consultations Using Advanced Medical Technology – Applications for NATO Operations», held in Zagreb, Croatia 13-16 September 2005

1. Introduction

Approximately 80,000 dependent pediatric patients reside in the Pacific area of responsibility, and Tripler Army Medical Center provides the pediatric subspecialty care for this population. Congenital heart disease affects approximately 1% of all live births, making abnormalities of the cardiovascular system the most common birth defect [1-2]. In addition, at least 90% of all pediatric patients will have a heart murmur detected at some point in their life, mostly innocent in nature [3-13]. From this large patient population, the primary care physician must quickly and accurately determine which patients require pediatric cardiology consultation at Tripler Army Medical Center. Unfortunately, multiple investigators have demonstrated poor auscultation skills among the primary care physicians tasked with the care of these children [14-17]. Taken together, the high prevalence of auscultatory findings and poor auscultation skills results in frequent evaluations of innocent heart murmurs, the most common reason for pediatric cardiology referral [10-11].

Currently, the pediatric cardiology division at Tripler Army Medical Center evaluates approximately 500 patients/yr with suspected heart disease from referral hospitals and clinics throughout the Pacific, some requiring air-evacuation of the patient and family members over great distances. These referrals for normal findings generate unnecessary costs and significant parental stress [18-19]. In contrast to primary care physicians, pediatric cardiologists can accurately diagnose the innocent heart murmur by auscultation alone, thereby eliminating the need for more costly studies [9-12]. Advances in electronic stethoscopy allow for the acquisition of digital heartsounds with transfer of these sounds to a computer for further evaluation and storage. This suggests the possibility of using digital heartsounds for telecardiology consultation, potentially eliminating the need to travel to the pediatric cardiologist. In two recent studies, pediatric cardiologists listening to recorded heartsounds were able to accurately diagnose innocent heart murmurs with a similar degree of accuracy when compared to traditional physical exam [20-21]. Taken together, these initial studies support the feasibility and reliability of remote pediatric heartsound interpretation.

The Pacific Asynchronous Tele-Health (PATH) system is an Internet based store-and-forward pediatric consultation system established in 2000 and is currently involved in successful diagnosis and management of numerous pediatric disease states. Using the PATH system, this project evaluated the ability to digitally acquire, electronically transfer, and accurately diagnose pediatric heartsounds as either normal or abnormal. In our study, echocardiographic validation was performed for all patients evaluated.

2. Methods

Institutional review board approval was obtained and all patients undergoing evaluation in the pediatric cardiology clinic at Tripler Army Medical Center were eligible for study enrollment. Each study subject underwent standard evaluation by a pediatric cardiologist (history, physical exam, and electrocardiogram) and complete echocardiography to establish a definitive cardiac diagnosis. Digital heartsound recordings, or phonocardiograms (PCGs), were acquired using a commercially available digital stethoscope attached to a handheld PDA (STG for Handheld, Stethographics Inc, Westborough, MA). Each participant had 20-second PCGs acquired from standard cardiac auscultation areas (aortic, pulmonic, tricuspid and mitral sites) while both upright and supine. Additionally, PCGs were obtained from each axilla and the mid-back in the upright position only. PCGs were stored as .wav files and digitally filtered via custom digital signal processing algorithms devised to mimic bell and diaphragm modes of a standard stethoscope. Filtered PCGs were then uploaded to the PATH telemedicine system following modifications to the file uploading protocols to allow multiple .wav files to be uploaded simultaneously. We developed a graphical user interface within the PATH telemedicine system to allow for playback in a manner similar to standard clinical auscultation (see figure 1). The PATH system automatically recognizes the .wav file name which corresponds to recording location, patient position, and filtration mode and places an icon on the chest diagram. By simply clicking on each of these icons, the PCG recorded from this chest wall site/patient position is automatically played using Windows© Media Player. The choice of Windows© Media Player, although somewhat limited in its ability to manipulate sound files and playback modes, was felt critical in that it is readily available and therefore allows for PCG playback on virtually any networked computer. We believe this will allow our system to be used in a wide variety of clinical settings. Three pediatric cardiologists, blinded to all other clinical information, evaluated each patient's PCG dataset and classified the case as either normal or pathologic. Evaluations based solely on PCG auscultation were compared to both clinical and echocardiographic results for each patient.

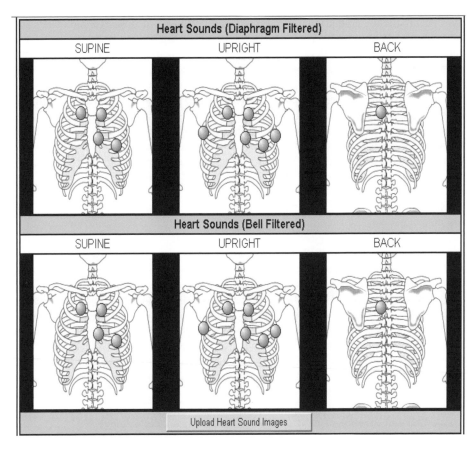

Figure 1. Graphical user interface allowing for simple playback of recorded heartsounds. When a red circle is selected, the corresponding phonocardiogram is automatically played using Windows© Media Player.

3. Results

Forty-one patients have been enrolled to date, each of which has been evaluated by all three pediatric cardiologists (total of 123 blinded PCG auscultation evaluations). Twenty-four patients had normal evaluations (16 with a normal auscultatory exam, 8 with an innocent murmur). The remaining seventeen patients had pathologic findings (table 1). All clinical diagnoses were confirmed by echocardiography, which revealed a tiny patent ductus arteriosus in one patient with no murmur. On average, each case was evaluated in 3-4 minutes using the PATH telemedicine system with the customized graphical user interface developed. Sound quality was rated as fair to good on most cases, with a rare report of poor sound quality. Of the 123 evaluations, 17 were misclassified as either normal/innocent versus pathologic, resulting in an overall accuracy of 86% (range of 81-90% among the three cardiologists). Of these seventeen, 8 cases were reported as normal/innocent murmur when pathology was present and 9 cases were evaluated as pathologic when actually normal/innocent murmur (sensitivity of 84%, specificity of 88%). Of the 8 with missed pathology, 5 errors of PCG auscultation evaluation could be attributed to two cases; one a tiny VSD (missed by all three pediatric cardiologists) and one case of partial anomalous pulmonary venous return (missed by 2/3 cardiologists). On retrospective, non-blinded review of the tiny VSD case, no murmur could be heard when listening to the PCG dataset; this murmur was very localized on clinical exam and the technician was not instructed to specifically record at this site (between the tricuspid and pulmonic area). The partial anomalous pulmonary venous return case was the second child enrolled in the study and the sound quality was suboptimal, most likely due us still learning the best methods to obtain high-quality recordings with little background noise. If these two cases are eliminated from the analysis for these technical considerations, overall accuracy of the system improves to 93% with a sensitivity of 94% and specificity of 88%. The other 3/8 pathologic cases deemed normal/innocent murmur missed by one cardiologist each were mild valvar pulmonary stenosis, mild right pulmonary artery stenosis, and one mitral stenosis with aortic insufficiency. Of those with normal/innocent murmur findings, 13% (9/72) were classified as pathologic. Of the innocent murmur cases, 92% were correctly identified (22/24).

4. Discussion

Using our PATH telemedicine system, with special modifications allowing upload and playback of recorded phonocardiograms, we were able to determine normal/innocent murmur from pathologic findings with a high degree of accuracy. Other investigators have demonstrated similar degrees of accuracy using a teleauscultation system for pediatric heart murmurs [20-21]. However, we believe our system offers the advantages of multiple recording sites, patient positions, and filtration modes as well as an easy to use graphical user interface that mimics actual clinical examination. We believe these are key features that can not only enhance accuracy but also improve acceptance of a teleauscultation system.

Since the major time and cost expenditure for remote patients is travel to our institution, we did not focus on making an actual diagnosis via telecardiology evaluation. Instead, we focused on determining normal/innocent from pathologic, since definitive diagnosis can be made at our site with our full array of diagnostic capabilities. One major benefit of such a system allows most patients with normal/innocent findings to be managed locally, without the need for travel to our institution for further evaluation. This can reduce healthcare expenditures, eliminate time away from work/duty station, and potentially reduce patient/family stress by providing more immediate diagnosis. Furthermore, patients with suspected pathologic lesions could be transferred more expeditiously, thereby improving time to diagnosis.

Our high degree of accuracy was achieved even with blinding of the cardiologist to all other clinical information. In clinical practice this would obviously not be the case, and we anticipate that the accuracy of the system will only improve when this clinical information is available. Furthermore, our recording protocol did not allow for modifications based on murmur location. As shown in our case with a tiny restrictive ventricular septal defect, this resulted in no murmur being recorded and hence was misinterpreted by all three cardiologist reviewers. In clinical practice the referring provider would surely guide the recording to include the findings in question, thereby improving overall accuracy of the system. Finally, there did seem to be an improvement in overall recording quality as we continued to enroll patients. Obtaining high-quality recordings in children, who are often not entirely cooperative, can be difficult. However, utilizing distraction (television with headphones), ambient noise reduction (turning off all electronic equipment in the recording lab), and comfortable patient positioning has resulted in higher quality PCGs. These simple and effective measures will be critical to the success of any teleauscultation projects.

Telecardiology evaluation must not be inferior to standard pediatric cardiology evaluation due to the risk of serious harm associated with heart disease mistakenly diagnosed as normal. In order to demonstrate the non-inferiority of our telecardiology approach, we will require a minimum of 90 patients to achieve statistical significance; for this reason we continue to enroll patients in the PacRim Pediatric Heartsounds Trial. Finally, we have begun to develop algorithms that automatically interpret PCGs using digital signal processing techniques. Our long-term goal is to incorporate these algorithms into the recording device itself, allowing for an immediate PCG interpretation at the bedside with physician overview as required.

Table 1. Pathologic diagnoses

Diagnosis	# patients
Restrictive ventricular septal defect	4
stenosis	4
Atrial septal defect/mitral regurgitation	2
Mitral stenosis/aortic insufficiency	2
Partial anomalous pulmonary venous return	1
Mild right pulmonary artery stenosis	1
Mitral valve prolapse	1
Pulmonary valve stenosis	1
Patent ductus arteriosus	1
TOTAL	17

References

[1] Ferencz C, Rubin JD, McCarter RJ, Brenner JI, Neill CA, Perry LW, et al. Congenital heart disease: prevalence at livebirth-the Baltimore-Washington infant study. Am J Epidemiol 1985;121:31-36.

[2] Samanek M, Slavik Z, Zborilova B, Hrobonova V, Voriskova M, Skovranek J. Prevalence, treatment, and outcome of heart disease in live-born children: a prospective analysis of 91,823 live-born children. Pediatr Cardiol 1989;10:205-211.

[3] van Oort A, Hopman J, de Boo T, van der Werf T, Rohmer J, Daniels O. The vibratory innocent heart murmur in schoolchildren: a case-control Doppler echocardiographic study. Pediatr Cardiol 1994;15:275-281.

[4] van Oort A, le Blanc-Botden M, de Boo T, van der Werf T, Rohmer J, Daniels O. The vibratory innocent heart murmur in schoolchildren: difference in auscultatory findings between school medical officers and a pediatric cardiologist. Pediatr Cardiol 1994;15:282-287.

[5] Rajakumar K, Weisse M, Rosas A, Gunel E, Pyles L, Neal WA, et al. Comparative study of clinical evaluation of heart murmurs by general pediatricians and pediatric cardiologists. Clin Pediatr 1999;38:511-518.

[6] McLaren MJ, Lachman AS, Pocock WA, Barlow JB. Innocent murmurs and third heart sounds in black schoolchildren. Br Heart J 1980;43:67-73.

[7] Bergman AB, Stamm SJ. The morbidity of cardiac nondisease in schoolchildren. N Engl J Med 1967;276:1008-1013.

[8] Fogel DH. The innocent systolic murmur in children: a clinical study of its incidence and characteristics. Am Heart J 1960;59:844-855.

[9] Newberger JM, Rosenthal A, Williams RG, Fellows K, Miettinen OS. Noninvasive tests in the initial evaluation of heart murmurs in children. N Engl J Med. 1983;308:61-64.

[10] McCrindle BW, Shaffer KM, Kan JS, Zahka KG, Rowe SA, Kidd L. Cardinal clinical signs in the differentiation of heart murmurs in children. Arch Pediatr Adolesc Med 1996;150:169-174.

[11] Smythe JF, Teixeira OHP, Vlad P, Demers PP, Feldman W. Initial evaluation of heart murmurs: are laboratory tests necessary? Pediatrics 1990;86:497-500.

[12] Geva T, Hegesh J, Frand M. Reappraisal of the approach to the child with heart murmurs: is echocardiography mandatory? Int J Cardiol 1988;19:107-113.

[13] Danford DA, Nasir A, Gumbiner C. Cost assessment of the evaluation of heart murmurs in children. Pediatrics 1993;91:365-368.

[14] Mangione S, Nieman L. Cardiac auscultatory skills of internal medicine and family practice trainees: a comparison of diagnostic proficiency. JAMA. 1997;278:717-722.

[15] Gaskin PRA, Owens SE, Talner NS, Sanders SP, Li JS. Clinical auscultation skills in pediatric residents. Pediatrics. 2000;105:1184-1187.

[16] Haney I, Ipp M, Feldman W, McCrindle BW. Accuracy of clinical assessment of heart murmurs by office based (general practice) paediatricians. Arch Dis Child. 1999;81:409-412.

[17] Vashist S, Shuper S. Clinical auscultation skills in pediatric residents. Pediatric Cardiology. 2002;23:668.

[18] Giuffre RM, Walker I, Vaillancourt S, Gupta S. Opening Pandora's box: Parental anxiety and the assessment of childhood murmurs. Canadian J Cardiology 2002;18:406-414.

[19] Geggel RL, Horowitz LM, Brown EA, Parsons M, Wang PS, Fulton DR. Parental anxiety associated with referral of a child to a pediatric cardiologist for evaluation of a Still's murmur. J Pediatrics 2002;140(6):747-752.

[20] Dahl LB, Hasvold P, Arild E, Hasvold T. Heart murmurs recorded by a sensor based electronic stethoscope and e-mailed for remote assessment. Arch Dis Child 2002;87(4):297-300.

[21] Belmont JM. Mattioli LF. Accuracy of analog telephonic stethoscopy for pediatric telecardiology. Pediatrics. 2003:112(4):780-6.

73

Remote Controlled Robot Performing Real-Time Echocardiography on Distance – a New Possibility in Emergency and Dangerous Areas

Mona OLOFFSON[a,b], Kurt BOMAN[a,b,c]

[a] *Department of Medicine, Skellefteå County Hospital*
[b] *HeartNet, Skeria, Skellefteå*
[c] *Department of Public Health and Clinical Medicine, Umeå University, Sweden*

Abstract. *Background:* Echocardiography is important in examining various cardiac conditions and, in particular to verify heart failure. It is seldom performed in a primary care centre (PHC) setting, especially not in sparsely populated areas.
Aim: To develop a concept that enables long-distance real-time echocardiography, preferably in rural PHCs.
Method: A robotic arm (Mobile Robotics AB, Skellefteå) has been developed to which an ultrasound probe is connected. A mobile ultrasound unit is placed at the patient's primary care site. A broadband link between the patient and the ultrasound operator is required in order to view the patient and the exact position of the probe, microphone, monitors and loudspeaker. The operator controls the robot and the ultrasound machine remotely with a joystick with the aid of newly developed software (Alkit Communication AB, Luleå). The ultrasound machine software is also remotely controlled by a virtual keyboard. Consultation between specialist, primary physician, operator and patient is done directly after the echocardiographic examination.
Result: Trials have been completed between the following locations: Luleå-Arvidsjaur (150 km), Umeå-Skellefteå (140 km) and Gothenburg-Skellefteå (1300 km). The procedure has provided satisfying results regarding long distance communication and image quality. However, more tests are necessary to evaluate patient satisfaction, cost-effectiveness and potential benefit for the health care system.
Conclusion: It is feasible to perform real-time echocardiography at a long distance by using present-day information technology (IT) and robotics. Echocardiography and specialist consultation with the patient can be done concurrently. In the future this concept might provide the opportunity for patients in rural areas to get rapid and accurate diagnosis and management of heart diseases.

This study was funded by: HeartNet, Skeria, Skellefteå, 931 86 Skellefteå, Sweden.
This study was presented at the advanced research workshop, NATO ARW, Zagreb, Sept 13-15, 2005

1. Introduction

The demographic situation is changing in the western societies with more elderly people who will need health care, nursing and rehabilitation. We also face new hospital structures, smaller but more specialised for acute treatment. In the future it is likely that more treatment and rehabilitation of patient will occur in their homes. There is a need to find new solutions for providing advanced diagnosis and disease management at a patient's home. One of these solutions may be newly developed information technology, services and products.

Chronic heart failure (CHF) affects about two percent of the general population with an increasing prevalence with age affecting approximately 10 percent of those over 75 years of age [1]. CHF is the only cardiovascular condition in which both the prevalence and incidence continue to rise [2]. CHF carries a high morbidity and is the leading cause of hospitalisation amongst those over 65 years of age [3]. The high morbidity and mortality rate is accompanied by a high cost for congestive heart failure management. The annual inpatient and outpatient expenditure on congestive heart failure in Sweden has been estimated at 2,6 billion Swedish crowns [4].

2. Background

Northern Sweden is characterised by an aging population with rising costs for maintaining current high levels of health care and affiliated social services. This also includes health care. In the late 1990's we started to focus on medical and social problems for CHF patients and the lack of coordination between health care providers, researchers, innovators and the medical industry. At that time there where few available commercial solutions utilizing current technology with its accompanying advantages. Priority was given to search for a solution that reduced this disadvantage of geographical distance for an aging population. In the county of Västerbotten, the public health care system was an early player in the area of telemedicine, partially owing to its high quality of broadband coverage. We brought together representatives for health care, a cardiologist and a sonographer within the framework of a European Union project called HeartNet. The project started in 2001 when potential partners were contacted for the purpose of developing solutions for these heart failure patients. Our idea was based on experiences from providing primary health care centres (PHC) with special expertise using an ordinary videoconference system and a portable echomachine. In 2001, clinical and scientific co-operation was started with PHC is in the counties of Västerbotten and Norrbotten, in northern Sweden. Beginning in 2002 we performed echocardiography with a portable echo-machine and video-consultation at the PHC, initially by visiting the health care centres, since 2003 videoconferencing has been used. In late 2002 the idea was born to develop a robot system in order to perform echocardiographic examination of heart patients at a distance. Through another EU-project, DITRA, contact was established with Alkit Communication, a company that develops and supplies technical support for advanced IT-communication. DITRA is a state of the art concept for video conferencing that offers the possibility of an interactivity application on the same platform. This advanced IT solution was named "the second generation telemedicine". Using this technique it is possible to support demanding clinical investigations at a distance. The reason for this second generation telemedicine was the need for high quality communications. It is based on the concept of a module based communication environment by utilizing the established broadband potentials with the aid of standard desktop computers. Another desired innovation was to enable a two-way transfer of patient information directly in the telemedicine situation. One great advantage is the combination of synchronous asynchronous communication. By this means it was possible to support regional development to move knowledge to the patient and to export top expertise services to surrounding regions in our catchment area.

3. The Telemedicine Concept

The goal was to develop and test a safe, efficient and dynamic electronic environment for communication and examination in order to improve quality of life for heart failure patients. More explicitly, to shorten time to diagnosis, reduce costs for the health care system and ease agony and suffering for patients by providing consultative opportunities. We also wished to develop new diagnostic algorithms for heart failure in PHC, especially the introduction of echocardiography. The robotic system was developed from an established industrial robot, but rebuilt to satisfy the highly qualified demands of a "medical robot" (Figure 1). Mobile Robotics constructed a mobile, remote controlled robotic arm that holds the transducer. We used a commercially available portable ultrasound machine, Cypress (Siemens AB). The robotic system, the portable ultrasound machine and web cameras are placed remotely at the PHC some distance from the cardiologist and the sonographer. The echocardiographic examination is performed by the sonographer, followed thereafter by a video conference between the general practitioner, the patient, the sonographer and the cardiologist. A schematic describes communication links and interactions between patient and provider (Figure 2).

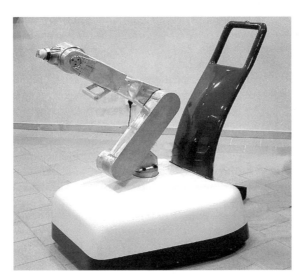

Figure 1. This picture shows the components and technical specifications for the Robotic system. A Mobile, Remote Controlled, Sonographer Support that holds the transducer during the ultrasound examination of a patient.

Channels of communication

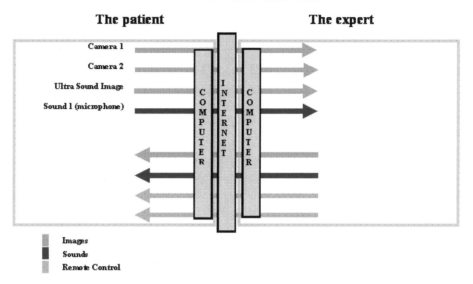

Figure 2. This is a schematic view of the telemedicine concept showing the cameras, ultrasound image, microphones and the remote control of the robotic arm and the echo machine

Another option was to find a system to improve the quality in the management process. We also wanted to improve therapy by optimising all kinds of treatment and finally our aim was to create new products and services.

This paper describes our early experience in testing the technical feasibility of this methodology, to provide cardiac echo consultation at distance.

4. Results

Robotic technology has been tested in several situations. Initial laboratory examinations with the robotic arm yielded satisfactory echocardiographic presentation and information. The first demonstration between two primary health care centres was performed in 2003 and revealed that this type of examination was possible with current broadband infrastructure with a satisfying image quality. Long distance examinations were performed within the county of Västerbotten and the county of Norrbotten. In 2004 we demonstrated the system at The Annual General Meeting of the Swedish Society of Medicine in Gothenburg. The ultrasound robot and communication platform were also presented for ministers of health at the EU-summit in Tromsö, Norway. This was the first international demonstration of the robot system.

5. The Potential for Application of Remote Control Echocardiography

Clinical applicability in remote rural areas with limited excess to cardiac expertise is obvious.Another important application for this system is a potential solution for ergonomic problems for sonographers. It is well known that many sonographers develop severe and chronic pain in their shoulders and neck from overuse. The robotic system offers the potential to reduce or eliminate this type of injury. We can also imagine special situations where this remote control echocardiographic system has many advantages such as battlefield situations and emergency areas. In these cases the remote control robot system could perform advanced diagnostic procedures from a centralized care facility. We can also see advantages of this system in ambulances, mobile health care systems and oil platforms and disaster situation when medical personnel may be exposed to hazardous such as chemicals, radiation or biological pollution.

6. Advantages with Telemedicine Consultation

Our impression is that this kind of system is useful in many ways. We have found that we could directly confirm or exclude heart failure cases. By using the video consultation system we could immediately discuss differential diagnoses, and of course, discuss different treatment proposals, including specialty referrals to specialized centres. Dialogue between the PHC and the specialist centre is an important feature of the system and includes the communication between the patient and the sonographer. This concept also affords an excellent opportunity for education of the general practitioner and shortens cardiologist consultation time.

7. Discussion

Our experience based on tests that have been performed to date with this robotic system in an experimental situation is feasible both in regional, national and international areas. This system has been used only in experimental situations and has thus far not been put into routine clinical practise. The aim of our telemedicine concept is to commence with cardiology consultation with the robotic system in the autumn 2005.There is a growing interest in telemedicine, but so far publications and reports on clinical results are somewhat sparse. Recently a study called TEN-HMS [5] compared different patient groups using telemedicine with promising results. They studied whether home telemonitoring (HTM) could improve outcomes compared with nurse telephone support (NTS) and usual care (UC) for patients with heart failure who were at high risk of hospitalization or death. They found that the number of admissions and mortality were similar among patients randomly assigned to NTS or HTM, but the mean duration of admissions was reduced by 6 days (95% confidence interval 1 to 11) with HTM. Patients randomly assigned to receive UC had higher one-year mortality (45%) than patients assigned to receive NTS (27%) or HTM (29%) ($p = 0.032$). They concluded that further investigation and refinement of the application of HTM are warranted because it may have a valuable role for the management of selected patients with heart failure [3].

As far as we know there is no system like ours for examining the heart at a distance and there are no publications so far on clinical studies by using a remote controlled robotic arm with echocardiography. However there have been experiences with different kinds of robot techniques for example the OTELO consortium [6] They used a tele-operated robotic chain for real-time ultrasound image acquisition and medical diagnosis primarily of the liver and kidney. They showed that they were able to identify 66% of lesions and 83% of symptomatic pathologies.

So far there are a number of unanswered questions about this technology. We know very little of satisfaction of patients participating in this kind of procedure. We also know very little how this system will work in practice in a health care system. There are also few data on the effects on morbidity and cost effectiveness, or if there is a more efficient use of specialist services. These questions have the highest priority in the future.

In conclusion, our experiences so far with a remote controlled echocardiography and IT have shown that this system is feasible in an experimental situation, both in a regional area and also in national and international areas. The system is now ready to be tested in real clinical situations. Aside from the need for clinical problem solving in remote and rural areas, there may be other important applications for this system such as a work solution for sonographers and use in dangerous areas like battlefield and emergency situations, chemically and bacteriologically contaminated areas, as well as X-ray contaminated areas.

References

[1]   Swedberg K, Cleland J, Dargie H, Drexler H, Follath F, Komajda M, et al. Guidelines for the diagnosis and treatment of chronic heart failure: executive summary (update 2005): The Task Force for the Diagnosis and Treatment of Chronic Heart Failure of the European Society of Cardiology. Eur Heart J, 2005;26(11):1115-40.

[2]   Yamani M, Massie BM. Congestive heart failure: insights from epidemiology, implications for treatment. Mayo Clin Proc, 1993,68(12):1214-8.

[3]   Graves EJ, Gilium BS. 1994 summary: National Hospital Discharge Survey. Adv. Data, 1996,278:1-12

[4]   Rydén-Bergsten, Andersson F. The health care cost in Sweden. J Intern Med, 1999, 3: 275-84.

[5]   Cleland JG, Louis AA, Rigby AS, Janssens U, Balk AH; TEN-HMS Investigators Noninvasive home telemonitoring for patients with heart failure at high risk of recurrent admission and death: the Trans-European Network-Home-Care Management System (TEN-HMS) study.J Am Coll Cardiol., 2005 May 17,45(10):1654-64.

[6]   Delgorge C, Courreges F, Al Bassit L, Novales C, Rosenberger C, Smith-Guerin N, Bru C, Gilabert R, Vannoni M, Poisson G, Vieyres P. A tele-operated mobile ultrasound scanner using a light-weight robot. IEEE Trans Inf Technol Biomed., 2005 Mar,9(1):50-8.

A Functional Telemedicine Environment in the Framework of the Croatian Healthcare Information System

Aljoša PAVELIN [b,e], Ivica KLAPAN [a,b,d], Mario KOVAČ [a,b,d], Milica KATIĆ [b,c,f],
Ranko STEVANOVIĆ [b,g], Mladen RAKIĆ [b,h], Nives KLAPAN [i]

[a] Telemedicine Committee, Ministry of Health and Social Welfare, Republic of Croatia
[b] Croatian Telemedicine Society, Croatian Medical Association, Zagreb, Croatia
[c] Committee for development of State program of health care and development of telemedicine on islands, Ministry of the Sea, Tourism, Transport and Development, Republic of Croatia
[d] Reference center of the Ministry of Health and Social Welfare for computerized surgery and telesurgery, Zagreb, Croatia
[e] Metronet telekomunikacije d.d, Sektor za mrežu i usluge, Zagreb, Croatia
[f] Department of Family Medicine, School of Public Health «Andrija Štampar», Zagreb, Croatia
[g] Croatian Institute for Public Health, Zagreb, Croatia
[h] Clinical Hospital Split, Department of Anesthesiology and Intensive Care, Split, Croatia
[i] Department of Telemedicine, Zagreb, Croatia

The paper was presented at the Advanced Research Workshop «Remote Cardiology Consultations Using Advanced Medical Technology – Applications for NATO Operations», held in Zagreb, Croatia 13-16 September 2005

"... integration, monitoring and management of patients, education of patient and staff using systems that can allow quick access to experts' consultation and patients' information, regardless of where patients or information may reside ..."
(1990., American Telemedicine Association, Washington D.C., USA.)
"Establishment of integrated national health information structure will enable an easy access to medical information for all of the citizens and at the same time medical professionals will be able to follow up on patients condition and provide medical services to patients located in distance and rural areas. Such health system should enable better medical prevention and treatments and result in reduction of health expenses and expenses related to sick leave."
(«Development strategy of Republic of Croatia in 21st century», «Croatia in 21st century – Information and communication technology », Working group of the Department for strategic development of Republic of Croatia)
'eHealth refers to the use of modern information and communication technologies to meet needs of citizens, patients, healthcare professionals, healthcare providers, as well as policy makers.' – from e-Health Ministerial Declaration 22 May 2003.

1. Introduction to Telemedicine

Health care service represents one of the pillars of every civilized society. It is implemented through the existing network of medical institutions on primary, secondary and third level. The quality of entire health system, among other things, depends on availability and timeliness of health care in rural areas where distance separates the patients from modern medical centers and therefore jeopardizes those patients additionally [1].By usage of modern telemedicine systems doctors on geographically dispersed locations, or within the same location, are able to communicate directly with patient and to consult mutually which enables them to share important medical information in any form.

By use of audio/visual communication and transmission of laboratory results, RTG, EKG, EEG, CT, MRI [2], and other medical information, telemedicine system enables care provider to make fast and reliable diagnoses and prescribe therapy. Quality visual contact with patient enables doctors experts/consultants to provide "distance examination" and provides fast and high quality care for patient. This is especially important in emergency cases when right and fast diagnose might be out of crucial importance for patient. Usage of telemedicine system will as well significantly decrease number of unnecessary engagements of expensive transportation vehicles like boats or helicopters, which in cases of bad weather conditions might not be available for help. So far completed economical studies for telemedicine projects in the world, show that medical care of this kind is cost-effective.

To doctors in distance and small medical centers this would enable contacts with leading experts of clinical medicine in Croatia and Europe and therefore provide great help for their research and scientific work. This would stop the fluctuation of medical stuff from home country and provide better conditions for development of medical care in general.

In the light of the above said, the telemedicine systems could significantly increase level of health care in total and make it faster and efficient as well as reduce expenses on a long-term basis. The realization plan for any integrated telemedicine system implies the implementation of video communication segment, which has to be developed in accordance with defined requirements of medical profession regarding system functionality [3].This plan should include the analysis for the existing situation and the step-by-step solution proposal for the telemedicine system, in the aspect of telemedicine equipment and connections, as well as the videoconference equipment. Special attention should be given to telecommunication structure of the system and required terminal equipment and connections. Technical characteristics and performances of entire equipment should be explained in details. During plan development process special attention should be given to finding economically acceptable solutions that would support high communication standards that any telemedicine system requires. Advantages that proposed communication segment brings to telemedicine system are flexibility and scalability. In this sense, the system must be entirely based on accepted international standards.

Therefore, when developing any work proposal for telemedicine integrated system, possibilities and framework for the future development and update of the system should be considered, with end goal of integrating the existing system in the general national integrated information system.

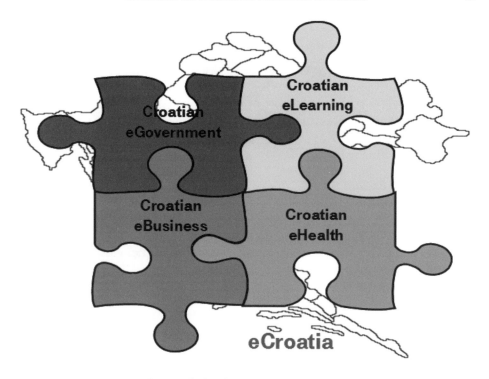

Figure 1. The Croatian eHealth within the eCroatia

2. Croatian eHealth - Croatian healthcare information system

The eEurope is a vision of information society for all that is built on four pillars – eGovernment, eLearning, eBusiness and eHealth. Within the e-Europe landscape, the e-Croatia is being born. Definition of a national information infrastructure [2] framework is a necessary prerequisite for the creation of the Croatian integrated information system – e-Croatia. Such well defined environment would significantly decrease the number of unjustified investments and abandoned projects by preventing uncoordinated activities and projects overlapping.

E-Croatia is the vision of new Croatian information society built on four pillars – e-Government, e-Business, e-Learning and e-Health (Fig.1). Definition of the national information infrastructure [1] based on contemporary information and communications technology is the key precondition for the creation of the e-Croatia. Croatian e-Health embraces institutions of primary and secondary healthcare as well as institutions for medical education.

Croatian e-health is foreseen to be an interactive establishment with soft borders but well defined interfaces. This should create a constructive virtual environment for correlation with other relevant national subjects such as Ministry of Health, Ministry of Science, Technology and Sports, Croatian Institute for Health Insurance, Search and Rescue Service (Fig. 2). Transparent interconnection with relevant international information systems would be enabled as well.

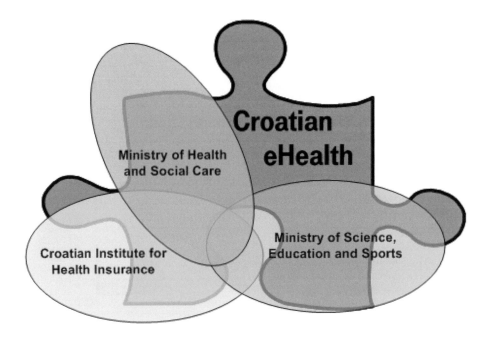

Figure 2. A Functional Environment of the Croatian eHealth

Key functional elements of the e-Health system are Telemedicine, Public Health Information and Administrative segments.

The Public Health Information segment should provide for public access to medical knowledge information and medical online services. The Internet is foreseen to be used for public access to healthcare information and services provided by the Croatian e-Health. The Administration segment includes all needed business applications and services ensuring normal functioning of the e-Health system.

3. Telemedicine Segment

Telemedicine segment is one of the building blocks of the e-Health system and therefore should be completely built upon the common underlying information infrastructure of the Croatian e-Health. The telemedicine is generally defined as the use of information and communications technologies (ICT) for transfer of medical information. More precisely, telemedicine activities include acquisition, processing, transmission and storage of medical data [3]. Real-time multimedia services are the essence of telemedicine and accomplish direct welfare for the patient and society as a whole.

Telemedicine equipment and applications provide means for remote consultations, diagnostics, surgery and education regardless the distance, increasing the overall healthcare quality. Real-time multimedia services are the essence of telemedicine and accomplish direct welfare for the patient and society as a whole. According to this, videoconference is the essential service to be implemented. The videoconference introduces interactivity into medical communications and provides physicians with crucial tool for adequate and timely reaction in emergency situations, in the same way as during normal medical activities [4].

Installed videoconferencing systems must fully comply with recognized standards and ensure acquisition, processing and transfer of the audio-visual information as well as data and static images. Built-in interfaces should be able to receive signals from personal computers, ECG, EEG, ultra sound, endoscope cameras and other sophisticated medical equipment and provide for high quality communications through ISDN and IP networks. When using such systems, it is possible to perform consultations and educate doctors, assist in operations [5] and diagnose independently of location and distance.

Interactivity is the main advantage of communication that is enabled by such systems since activities can only be coordinated and corrected in real time. Thanks to the interactive nature of communication, necessary technical preconditions for timely and qualitative reactions in crisis situations are ensured for the doctor

4. The eHealth Information and Communications Technology Platform

The Information Technology (IT) revolution stimulated by the Internet has resulted in deleting, what used to be solid, borders between almost all human professions. This has resulted in need for development of the universal information platform on global level that would enable the transmission of information in any form. Basic characteristics of a global information platform are universal communication platform, multimedia services and open approach. Each of the above mentioned characteristics have its own uniqueness that need to be harmonized. The Croatian eHealth with its telemedicine segment would function as a part of such converged environment. In that sense, majority of legality from global information area is transferred into defined telemedicine segment.

Real-time multimedia services are essence of telemedicine. Because of this, services and applications focused on benefits of patients and public in general would be implemented within the telemedicine segment. The benefits for patients are achieved through consultations, diagnostics, practice and education and the benefits for public in general are achieved through functional and financial efficacy, which contributes to overall civilization progress.

In the part of administrative functioning the telemedicine segment would continue on the existing resources of the health information system. Those resources understand installed equipment and implemented applications that are enabling functioning of the health system in general.

Communications platform of the telemedicine segment, by means of infrastructure, is the unique platform of the overall Croatian eHealth system. This platform must be standards-based. Built-in networking mechanisms would virtually partition Croatian eHealth on telemedicine, administrative, public access and other anticipated logical segments. Use of adequate network technology and mechanisms would create technical preconditions for the implementation of real-time services such as videoconference and IP Telephony. Technical preconditions understand offered Quality of service (QoS) level by means of guaranteed bandwidth, delay, jitter and packet loss for targeted flows of real-time traffic.

From the architectural perspective, the e-Health communications platform would follow hierarchical, 3-layer architecture. Dispersion of network functionalities across access, distribution and core layers would ensure network efficiency and reliability. Physically, e-Health system will be formed of a number of Local Area Networks (LAN) integrated into an intranet, by means of Wide Area Network (WAN) resources leased from telecom operator/service provider. This hierarchical network architecture ensures simplicity, fault-isolation and security, but most importantly it facilitates e-Health system upgrades and scaling.

In order to build an efficient and highly-performing communication infrastructure, traffic demands of implemented applications should be precisely determined. Analytical methods and software tools need to be used for determination of traffic patterns and needed QoS parameters [3]. Calculated results will be exploited in order to define network architecture, plan network resources, choose proper networking technology and equipment, and implement QoS and security mechanisms.

Openness of the Croatian e-Health is its strength, but introduces certain security issues. Security is not an ICT element. It must be observed as an ever evolving process that embraces the e-Health system at all levels – from physical access to facilities to data encryption. Security policy needs to be clearly defined, strictly implemented, proactively monitored and constantly adjusted. Conformance to international standards and regulations such as HIPAA (Health Insurance Portability and Accountability Act) and BS7799 is mandatory.

5. LAN Segment

LAN segment architecture would be adjusted to four anticipated cases; small practice, medium-size practice, one-building hospital and hospital campus. Depending on particular case L2 or L3 switches would be installed in the access layer. Distribution layer would be built of L3/L4 switches which provide for advanced networking functionalities. LAN platform would be based on Fast Ethernet (IEEE802.3u) and Gigabit Ethernet (IEEE 802.3ab and IEEE 802.3z) technologies.

LAN core layer would be formed in cases of technically justified need. Core layer would be completely based on fiber optic media. Depending on particular location characteristics and distances, Metro Ethernet concept with Gigabit Ethernet (IEEE 802.3z) technology would provide for an advanced solution. It is anticipated that such need will presumably arise in large towns like Zagreb, Split, Rijeka and Osijek. Link and equipment redundancy at distribution and core layers is mandatory.

Wireless LAN (WLAN), technology can be deployed inside controlled environments of medical institutions and it is acceptable for administrative purposes and general public services. Confidential data and patient-critical, real-time traffic should be kept within the cable segment.

6. WAN Segment

WAN segment of the Croatian eHealth should be built on network resources leased from a telecom/service provider (Fig. 3) This will considerably decrease initial investment (Capital Expenditures) as well as operational costs (Operational Expenditures). VPN concept based on IP/MPLS (Internet Protocol/Multi Protocol Label Switching) technology would provide for high level of flexibility and scalability. This concept also ensures fairly high level of initial security to user's traffic. Described VPN concept is

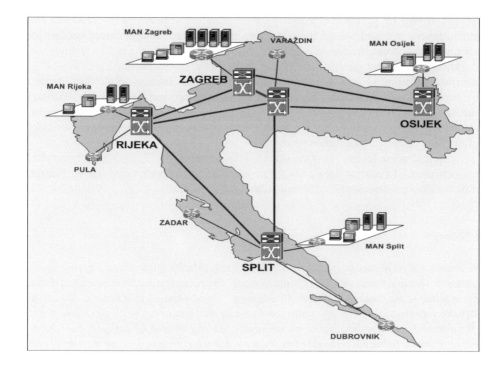

Figure 3. The Croatian eHealth Communications Platform

therefore presumed as a logical choice for WAN realization. In addition, this concept facilitates seamless merging with related information systems within the eCroatia as well as outside Croatian national space when required. Through the prism of globalization trends this is a relevant feature.

7. Remote Access Segment

Mobile subjects of the Croatian eHealth such as Emergency Response (ER) and search and rescue services during field intervention, and physicians at home or on travel will need access to internal eHealth resources. In order to enable such remote access any implemented access technologies can be used, including POTS (Plain Old Telephone Service), ISDN (Integrated Services Digital Network), ADSL (Asymmetric Digital Subscriber Line) and GPRS (General Packet Radio Service). Ongoing activities on implementation of national UMTS (Universal Mobile Telecommunications System) network will significantly mitigate limitations of audio-visual information wireless transfer.

8. IT Support

IT support will be provided through the administrative segment of the eHealth. The administrative segment would include hardware, software and personnel needed for governing and administration support.

Hardware implies generic servers like mail, www, DNS, and databases as well as specific application servers. Software implies appropriate business applications needed for every-day operations like administration, accounting, and procurement. Distinct care should be taken when purchasing or developing such applications. Standardized and widely adopted solutions that enable transparent implementation into broader information environments should be chosen.

Required prerequisite for successful implementation of IT support is continued reorganization of Croatian public healthcare system and comprehensive standardization of its business processes, and documentation.

9. Security

As already stated in part 4., openness of the Croatian eHealth emphasizes security issues. Common security threats in today's networking environments include viruses, Trojans and worms, spam, packet sniffers, IP spoofing , man-in-the-middle attacks, Denial of Service, various application level attacks. These threats can severely disrupt clinical and administrative business processes, consequently leading to loss of patients, confidence and significant financial costs.eHealth security must be observed as an ever evolving process, hence defined security policy and implemented mechanisms must be constantly adjusted. A comprehensive approach to information protection must be taken at every potential access point on all eHealth levels. Recognition of potential threats and access points would be the initial step in creating a secure environment. Next step assume implementation of appropriate network security tools. These include antivirus packages, security agents, AAA (Authentication, Authorization and Accounting) services, dedicated network security devices (firewall, IPS, IDS) and encryption. Only careful planning, precise definition of a security policy, strict enforcement and proactive monitoring may produce needed level of security [1]. Staff education must be carried out constantly.

10. CPME Guidelines for Development of Telemedicine (Comité Permanent des Médecins Européens-CPME)

Criteria's adopted by Telemedicine Committee of the Ministry of Health and Social Welfare of Republic of Croatia (2003. year), Croatian Association for Telemedicine (2002. year) and Organization for Telemedicine, Zagreb (2003. year), as criteria's for development of modern telemedicine, are general technological, developing, legal and ethical guidance regarding implementation and usage of telemedicine in telecare, so called CPME Guidance for Telemedicine (CPME 97/033 - CPME 2001/112) defined by Standing Committee of European Doctors (Comité Permanent des médecins Européens).

In 1999 year the World Medical Association (WMA) has adopted ethical standpoints regarding telemedicine (CPME 97/033) defined by the Standing Committee of European Doctors (Comité Permanent des médecins Européens-CPME; CPME Guidance for Telemedicine CPME). It is recommended that the national medical associations of EU adopt ethical guidance for development of telemedicine.

General guidance for development conception of telemedicine are: a) transmission/storage of video and audio records in real time on the highest level, b) transmission/storage of images records and other medical data (EKG, UZV, EEG, laboratory results, tele-examinations of patients) on the highest level, c) maximum data protection, d) reliability and safeness of data transmission.

According to CPME guidance, telemedicine based on e-mail correspondence (Internet) should be used in doctor-patient communication only as a supplement to, and not as a replacement for "face-to-face" consultation. Therefore, all of the complicated communication messages that may be difficult to understand in doctor-patient relation and require personal contact/communication, information that may be negative to the patient or any messages which otherwise require personal follow up or support by doctor, should preferably be given person to person or by more advanced forms of telemedicine.

Therefore the CPME-guidance has recommended uses of e-mail communication in telemedicine in following cases: communication about laboratory results, follow-up of chronic disease patients, health promotion, administrative matters update (such as making an appointment). The security of e-mail telemedicine (*per viam* Internet) cannot be provided on an entirely safe basis. This should be acknowledged by all patients involved and safety improving protocols must be discussed with the patients and with other parties involved in telemedicine activities. The reasons for this, according to CPME guidance, are risks that might arise when using e-mail in health care and all of the participants in Internet telemedicine should be aware of such risks. Examples are: lack of integrity in original data, interruption of e-mail, destruction of data (intentional or unintentional) caused by various reasons, question of confidentiality, lack of identification of the patient as well as possible lack of liability insurance coverage. One of the additional problems that might rise during telemedicine practice is problem related to cross-border practice of medicine (one of bigger problems in EU).

The patients should, with no exceptions, be informed about the technical aspects and security of e-mail correspondence, and give their written consent (CPME 2001/112 Final Annex 2.). As well, patients should give their consent for any form of applied telemedicine.

11. Applying / implementing telemedicine

Applying such a developed telemedical system offers an exceptional advantage for growth, not only of mentioned medical centers, the entire Croatian medical supply, but also in providing/offering telecare to citizens of neighboring regions and entire countries.

Through this, all the mentioned medical centers become expert medical centers, not only in Croatia, but also in the region of southeast Europe, in offering expert/consultant tele-medical services [7,8,9].

Apart from this, the mentioned Croatian expert medical centers also become respectable "opinion leaders" for a large medical community in this part of Europe and leading centers in this entire region for the needs of developing modern telecare.

12. Expected Positive Results of the Initiated Telemedical Project

I. The planning and development of services

- Development of university hospital/business ''tele-practice''[10],
- Establishing multidisciplinary teams,
- New projects/management in tele-care,
- Refreshing knowledge, interviewing, counseling,
- Expanding and gaining new markets and users.

II. Training and education

- Professional and scientific university courses, upgrading,
assistance in ''in-Service'' training/upgrading, refreshing knowledge and skills

III. Basic telemedical communication

- consultations ''at a distance'', cardiology, rheumatology, dermatology, gynecology, radiology, neurology, pediatrics, psychiatry, orthopedics, oncology, ORL, ophthalmology, gastroenterology, stomatology, emergency medicine and others,
- access to ''inaccesible'' places, especially islands,
- ''presence'' of a specialist in rural areas, especially on islands,
- expertise before and during operations [11,12,13,14], post-operative consultations, medical support for special events

IV. Savings

- travel expenses (e.g. islands-coast/mainland of Croatia)
- call-center expertise,
- professional service for far-away, small medical centers, especially on islands
- improving health care for domestic and foreign citizens,
- improving the financial status of employees (financing of expert tele-services),
- immediate tele-service,
- diagnostic and therapy confirmed by expert/experts.

    The possible interest of the Ministry of health and social welfare in the Republic of Croatia for the implementation of proposed guidelines of a modern telemedical project

- Control and coordination of telemedical activities in Croatian health care, but in the future, in neighboring countries also
- Drafting of a detailed plan and programme of common rights and obligations between experts-consultants and doctors that require medical expertise, university hospital institutions that are a part of the telemedical network, Croatian Health Insurance Fund patients themselves
- Precise following and archiving of telemedical activities in all medical work places involved in this type of medical care
- Periodic evaluation of certain expert's and university hospital institution's work (professional-medical, economic, legal); monthly, bi-annually, annually

- Improving medical care of citizens in far-away and dislocated places (e.g. dislocated community health centers); professional-medical and economic indicators
- Improving the work of medical staff in smaller community health centers; professional-medical and economic indicators
- Implementing modern technology in everyday routine medical care [15]
- In this, Croatia would align itself with the more developed countries, as a country that keeps abreast of and implements modern technology in medical care of its population and foreign citizens (business people and the like)
- Realizing the development and implementation of modern technologies in the medical profession, with the goal to diagnose and treat patients in a quality manner and develop the medical science and expertise in a faster and purposeful manner
- Consultations/managing operations / tele-surgery (e.g. minimal invasive endomicrochirurgy for the nose and sinuses, functional and esthetic head operations etc.), that has already been performed in many instances from Zagreb (e.g. ORL University hospital Šalata/UHC Zagreb, University hospital for traumatology Zagreb, University hospital for surgery General Hospital „Sv.Duh") with UH Osijek/ORL [13,14], many times with community health center Makarska, General hospital Nova Bila/Bosnia and Herzegovina, etc.).

13. The importance of telemedicine in primary health care on islands

The island inhabitants, more than any other inhabitants in Croatia, use primary care. This can be concluded from the higher than average number of annual visits to doctors, especially house calls. For example, on Mljet 25% of all visits took place in patient's home [6].

According to the data on using primary health care in the narrow sense (service for family medicine and primary health care for preschool children), 84% of registered island inhabitants used health care.

In relation to other areas in Croatia, island inhabitants visit primary health care doctors more frequently, which is noticeable in a higher annual rate of doctors visits per island user (8,6 visits per patient for the islands, and 7,4 visits per patient for the mainland). The average number of referrals for specialist consultations per patient is the same, both for the mainland and for the islands, amounting to 1,6.

A more rational and purposeful referring can be achieved through teleconsultations, thus by applying it to island medicine, the quality of health care would improve, both for its citizens and for tourists while, at the same time, it would decrease the number of referrals for specialist consultations. According to professional evaluations of public health experts, the number of unnecessary specialist consultations would decrease 20%. Thus, the conclusion is that after establishing a teleconsultation system, 20% of all specialist consultations will be performed as teleconsultations.

Therefore, mutual consultations enable the most effective use of a doctor's expert knowledge in continuously and fully caring for patients and that of a specialist consultant.

Teleconsultation/telediagnostics on Croatian islands enables:

- The establishment of personal communication between doctors and consultants
- A doctor who refers patient to organize patients according to problems and illnesses and perform consultations for several patients at the same time
- Mutual consultations ("real time consultations», that is, consultations in real time)
- Relieving patients of the need to travel, loose time, take a day off from work, and at the same time, offer more quality care
- Assist the primary health care doctor in emergency, life-threatening conditions, especially doctors who work in isolated and hard to reach, or badly connected places (islands or far-away villages on the mainland)
- The patient or healthy visitor to be assured that, if the need arises, he/she would have access to specialist consultations no matter where they are located, or have consultations with his/her own doctor/doctors. This is especially significant for the development of health tourism and for designing the entire tourist programme.

Along with other professional preconditions, the confidentiality of data has to be absolutely protected in teleconsultations. The expected advantage of teleconsultations is in reducing unnecessary specialist consultations, performing more quality consultations and in the educative value of consultations both for doctors who refer patients and for consultants [6],especially in cardiology [16].

Upon establishing the teleconsultation system, it can be expected that 20% of all specialist consultations will be performed as teleconsultations [6].In conclusion, teleconsultations/telediagnostics in island medicine could significantly contribute to the quality of health care of the local population and tourists.

14. The Possible Interest of the Ministry of Sea. Tourism, Transport and Development in the Republic of Croatia for the Proposed Telemedical Project

- This type of telemedical care offers all tourists, business people (even though they will most often not use it at all), according to need, the possibility of contacting a doctor from their own region, and in that way directly influence the significant improvement in the economic and tourist programmes, that is rare anywhere else in the world.
- The Republic of Croatia will be recognized as a safe economic/tourist destination that is capable of providing additional tele-medical exams and consultations to all entrepreneurs/business people/tourists
- Increasing safety in the category of health care represents Croatia's attention to caring for its foreign and local guest, and as such, will surely be recognized
- On this telemedical basis, tourism can be developed all year round, for example in the category of climate spas (insufficiently developed until now) intended for treatment/care of chronic illnesses/patients. This means of caring for their health, due to the nature of their illness they belong to the patients that are at risk, for example cardiologic, would present and additional reason

for tour-operators to choose Croatia as a destination (tourist/medical) where to take their clients. In this, our spas would achieve their full meaning, since it has been proved that many of them have ideal climatic conditions for the above mentioned purposes

- An ideal opportunity to extend the tourist season is offered, more persons will be employed, significant economic development for the region, but also for Croatia as a whole, which certainly presents a special interest to the Ministry of Economy and to the Government of the Republic of Croatia
- Once The Croatian Tourist Board and the Ministry of Sea, Tourism, Transport and Development of the Republic of Croatia, accept and support this plan of developing the telemedical project as part of the implementation strategy of IT and communication technologies in the health care system [17], they can immediately enter the demanding world tourist market with a programme of a new and original tourist-medical product. This can surely influence the increase in the number of guests, especially those that are more demanding.

15. Standardization, Economics and Legislative Aspects

The simplification of the organization structure and business processes is unambiguous trend in all business systems of today. The goal of such changes is aimed at increasing business efficiency and decreasing the spending of time and funds.

Comprehensive activities on standardization [17] of organizational structure and business processes need to be carried out, throughout creation of the Croatian eHealth. Accordingly, a certain restructuring in the existing public health care system must be undertaken. Standardization enforcement in organizational structure, business procedures and documentation would significantly increase the overall system efficiency [2]. Furthermore, transparent binding with other information systems would be alleviated.

Design and implementation of the Croatian eHealth is a demanding, but feasible task. Not surprisingly, financial issues represent the key challenge. Besides Croatian government, related ministries and public services, manufacturers of ICT equipment and applications should be involved. Their interest and means for Return on Investment (RoI) should be based on proper functioning of the Croatian eHealth. Expenditures decrease should be observed as a long-term category, through simplification of business processes, increase in productivity and efficient reallocation of resources. Creating a public health information system, especially introducing the telemedicine segment, would bring about an increase in the quality and availability of medical services and cut back on time needed to react. The decrease in operational expenses should be viewed through a reduction in the number of unnecessary transports and hospitalization and as an increase of the creative time of medical staff.

Ongoing worldwide introduction of information systems into multilayered social environments opens up a number of regulatory issues that all modern societies need to answer. For example, the decision/proposal of where possible court cases could take place (city/country where the patient or doctor lives) due to negligence in telecare is still not defined in CPME Guidance for Telemedicine CPME (Comité Permanent des médecins Européens-CPME). Thereby, clear juridical platform represents a strategic stronghold in the eHealth creation process as well. The Republic of Croatia has to create a constructive juridical framework through legislative acts and regulations that will support development and operation of the eHealth and eCroatia as a whole. Common sense dictates utilization of international experience in this area, appropriate adjustment and implementation in the national framework.

16. Conclusion

Creation of the Croatian eHealth system, and particularly its Telemedicine segment, would significantly raise the quality and availability of medical services as well as shorten the time of reaction.

Croatian medicine will become a unique promoter of a special medical offers among domestic and foreign population in Croatia, users of medical services in neighboring countries, foreign travel agencies and insurance houses, from the most basic telemedical activities to modern telesurgical processes assisted by computers [19,20,21,22].

Despite actual obstacles at essential level in the Croatian public healthcare system and society as a whole, advisability of creating the healthcare information system – eHealth is doubtless and represents an evolutionary step. Telemedicine segment is anticipated as a crucial element that will serve as a foundation for development of the Croatian eHealth as a whole.

References

[1]   Afrić W, Bonačić J, Božić V, Čagalj M, Matošić N, Višić J. Komunikacijski sustav Službe hitne medicinske pomoći Županije splitsko-dalmatinske – HITNET. Book "Telemedicina u Hrvatskoj" (ed. Klapan I, Čikeš I), Medika 2001.
      Bešenski N, Pavić D. : Teleradiology. Book „Telemedicine" (ed. Klapan I, Čikeš I), Telemedicine Association Zagreb, 2005.

[2]   Carić L. : Telemedicine and IT system securiry. Book „Telemedicine" (ed. Klapan I, Čikeš I), Telemedicine Association Zagreb, 2005.

[3]   Ferek-Petrić B, Čikeš I. : Telemedicine in pacing. Book „Telemedicine" (ed. Klapan I, Čikeš I), Telemedicine Association Zagreb, 2005.

[4]   Feussner H, Ungeheuer A, Etter et al. : The potential of telecommunication in surgery. Langenbecks Arch Chir 1996; 2:525-527.

[5]   Jaramaz B. CAS in orthopedics. Book „Telemedicine" (ed. Klapan I, Čikeš I), Telemedicine Association Zagreb, 2005.

[6]   Katić M. : Teleconsultations in primary healthcare. Book „Telemedicine" (ed. Klapan I, Čikeš I), Telemedicine Association Zagreb, 2005.

[7]   Klapan I, Šimičić Lj, Kubat M, Strinović D. : Computer assisted FESS. 3rd EUFOS, editors: O.Ribari, A.Hirschberg, Monduzzi Editore, Bologna, str. 273-276, 1996.

[8]   Klapan I, Šimičić Lj, Rišavi R, Janjanin S. : Tele-3D-Computer Assisted Functional Endoscopic Sinus Surgery (Tele-3D-C-FESS). CARS'99 (ed. Lemke HU, Vannier MW, Inamura K, Farman AG), Elsevier, Amsterdam, N.York, Oxford, Shannon, Singapore,Tokyo, str. 784-789, 1999.

[9]   Klapan I, Rišavi R, Šimičić Lj, Simović S. : Tele-3D-C-FESS Approach with High-Quality Video Transmisstion. Otolaryngology Head Neck Surgery, 121 (2):P187-188, 1999.

[10] Klapan I, Vranješ Ž, Rišavi R, Šimičić Lj. Computer-assisted surgery and telesurgery in otorhinolaryngology. Book „Telemedicine" (ed. Klapan I, Čikeš I), Telemedicine Association Zagreb, 2005.

[11] Klapan I, Pavelin A. : Hrvatski Integrirani Telemedicinski Sustav. Videokomunikacije za potrebe telemedicinskog sustava. Book "Telemedicina u Hrvatskoj" (ed. Klapan I, Čikeš I), Medika 2001.

[12] Klapan I, Šimičić Lj, Rišavi R. : Tele-3D- Kirurgija potpomognuta računalom. Televirtualna kirurgija u realnom vremenu. Book "Telemedicina u Hrvatskoj" (ed. Klapan I, Čikeš I), Medika 2001.

[13] Klapan I, Šimičić Lj. : Telemedicine assisted surgery: Tele-3D-Computer assisted surgery in Rhinology. Telemedicine e-Health, 8(2):217, 2002.

[14] Klapan I, Šimičić Lj, Rišavi R, Pasarić K, Sruk V, Schwarz D, Barišić J. : Real-Time transfer of live video images in parallel with 3D modeling of the surgical field in computer-assisted telesurgery. J Telemed Telecare, 8:125-130, 2002.

[15] Klapan I, Šimičić Lj, Rišavi R, Bešenski N, Pasarić K, Gortan D, Janjanin S, Pavić D, Vranješ Ž. : Tele-3D-Computer Assisted Functional Endoscopic Sinus Surgery: new dimension in the surgery of the nose and paranasal sinuses. Otolaryngol Head Neck Surg, 12:325-334, 2002

[16] Kos M, Pavelin A, Buzolić J. : Računalna i telekomunikacijska osnovica telemedicine. Book "Telemedicina u Hrvatskoj" (ed. Klapan I, Čikeš I), Medika 2001.

[17] Kovač M. Efficient management of medical images. Book „Telemedicine" (ed. Klapan I, Čikeš I), Telemedicine Association Zagreb, 2005.

[18] Lam D, Poropatich R, Gilbert GB. Telemedicine standardization in the NATO environment. Book „Telemedicine" (ed. Klapan I, Čikeš I), Telemedicine Association Zagreb, 2005.

[19] Lončarić S. Virtual reality in medicine. Book „Telemedicine" (ed. Klapan I, Čikeš I), Telemedicine Association Zagreb, 2005.

[20] Miličić D, Čikeš I. : Telemedicina u kardiologiji. Book "Telemedicina u Hrvatskoj" (ed. Klapan I, Čikeš I), Medika 2001.

[21] Mauher M. : Telemedicina u okviru implementacijske strategije informacijske i komunikacijske tehnologije (ICT) u sustavu zdravstva Republike Hrvatske. Book "Telemedicina u Hrvatskoj" (ed. Klapan I, Čikeš I), Medika 2001.

[22] Pavelin A, Klapan I, Katić M, Klapan N. Croatian telemedicine program: active multilateral cooperation in telecare development in the 21st century. Book „Telemedicine" (ed. Klapan I, Čikeš I), Telemedicine Association Zagreb, 2005.

[23] Petrović-Zozoli J. : Elements of the preinvestment study of the investment in the "Adriatic-tele-doc" project". Book „Telemedicine" (ed. Klapan I, Čikeš I), Telemedicine Association Zagreb, 2005.

[24] Poropatich R, Morris TJ, Gilbert GR, Abbott KC. The US Army program for development telemedicine. Book „Telemedicine" (ed. Klapan I, Čikeš I), Telemedicine Association Zagreb, 2005.

[25] Satava RM. : Telesurgery - acceptability of compressed video for remote surgical proctoring - invited commentary. Arch Surg 1996; 131: 401.

[26] Schlag PM, Engelmurke F, Zurheyde MM, Rakowsky S, Graschew G. :Teleconference and telesurgery. Chirurg 1998; 69:1134-1140.

[27] Schwarz D, Barišić J. : Telesurgery. Book „Telemedicine" (ed. Klapan I, Čikeš I), Telemedicine Association Zagreb, 2005.

[28] Stevanović R, Klapan I. Establishment and development of e-Health information system in transitional countries (Croatian experience). Book „Telemedicine" (ed. Klapan I, Čikeš I), Telemedicine Association Zagreb, 2005.

[29] Šesto M, Batinić Z, Trbović A. Telemedciine in cardiology. Book „Telemedicine" (ed. Klapan I, Čikeš I), Telemedicine Association Zagreb, 2005.

[30] Šimičić Lj, Klapan I, Simović S, Brzović Z, Vukoja M, Rišavi R, Gortan D. : Computer assisted functional endoscopic sinus surgery. Video texture mapping of 3D models. E.R.S. and I.S.I.A.N., Wienna, Austria, (H. Stammberger, G. Wolf), Monduzzi Editore, Bologna, str. 281-285, 1998.

[31] Vuković-Obrovac J, Obrovac K. : DICOM standard of medical imaging data. Book „Telemedicine" (ed. Klapan I, Čikeš I), Telemedicine Association Zagreb, 2005.

Telemedicine Standardization in the NATO Environment

David LAM[a], Ronald K. POROPATICH[b], Gary R. GILBERT[c]

[a] *Charles McC. Mathias National Study Center for Trauma and Emergency Medical Systems, Baltimore Maryland, and U.S. Army Telemedicine and Advanced Technology Research Center, Fort Detrick Maryland*
[b] *Walter Reed Army Medical Center, Washington, D.C., and U.S. Army Telemedicine and Advanced Technology Research Center, Fort Detrick Maryland*
[c] *Department of Electrical Engineering, School of Engineering, University of Pittsburgh, Pittsburgh, PA , and U.S. Army Telemedicine and Advanced Technology Research Center, Fort Detrick Maryland*

Abstract. As the North Atlantic Treaty Organization has evolved its doctrine from that of strictly national medical support during operations to that of multinational medical support, the importance of, and the need for, Telemedicine standardization has become apparent. This article describes the efforts made by NATO in recent years to begin the process of Telemedicine (TMED) standardization within the Alliance.

The paper was presented at the Advanced Research Workshop «Remote Cardiology Consultations Using Advanced Medical Technology – Applications for NATO Operations», held in Zagreb, Croatia 13-16 September 2005.

1. NATO Background

During the cold war, the North Atlantic Treaty Organization's (NATO's)forces were lined up essentially shoulder to shoulder along the inter-German border. Each force was logistically self-sufficient, and interaction between these various corps was planned to be limited except along the corps boundaries. Logistics (including medical support) was considered to be a strictly national responsibility. Each nation planned to provide its own medical support to the maximum extent possible, from the front lines back to the home country. Nations deploying their forces over long distances (particularly the United States and Canada) did plan to make use of some host nation medical support in the countries they deployed through, but once in combat, they too planned strictly national medical systems.

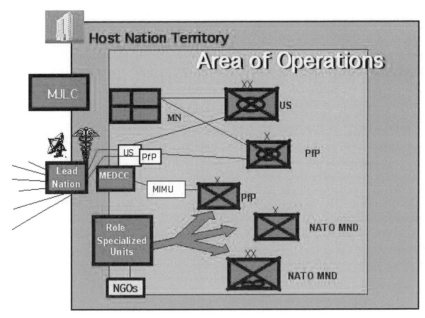

MEDCC= Medical Coordination Cell; MIMU= Multinational Integrated Medical Unit;
MJLC= Multinational Joint Logistic Center; MN= Multinational Unit; MND=
Multinational Division;NGO= Non-Governmental Organisations; PfP= Partnership
For Peace

Figure 1. New Conceptual Medical Force Laydown

When the Soviet Union collapsed, NATO developed a new concept of defence which affected medical support. No longer was the primary threat considered to be Soviet tank armies thundering into Germany, but regional instability, with failed states in NATO's area of interest, along with increased requirements for humanitarian support, disaster relief, and peace-keeping operations. Complicating this scenario was the demand on the part of the populations of the NATO nations for a "peace dividend", which led to rapid down-sizing of military forces in all the Alliance nations.

To deal with this new scenario, NATO developed several new concepts of operations. These concepts require new medical support structures and policies. No longer can each nation plan to "go it alone". Sharing of resources and multinationality has become the goal. But medical support in operations may be very complex [10]. Future medical support will entail: enhanced sustainment of optimal performance; increasing medical priorities for force protection, disease prevention and treatment of non-battle injuries; forward treatment only as necessary; rapid long-range evacuation; and medical informatics / telemedicine embedded throughout the spectrum of a health care system, including care for multi-national military and paramilitary forces as well as civilian non-combatants. In addition to some strictly national structures and capabilities, NATO anticipates an increased use of multinational support. Increased coordination with other multinational organizations and with private non-governmental organizations will be a necessity. [7] (Figure 1).

The increased use of multinational medical support is not simply a theoretical concept. It has actually been implemented during NATO operations in the former Yugoslavia during the past 8 years. In the Balkans, NATO forces are medically supported on a multinational basis, and it is not uncommon for soldiers of one nationality to be provided medical care in a medical facility operated by another nation, or even by a multi-national consortium. (Figures 2 and 3).

The cold war concept of moving large medical contingents to the battlefield, along with every type of subspecialization, is obviously no longer tenable in this new operational (and political) situation. Each nation participating in these operations has struggled with mechanisms to reduce the medical "footprint" in the operational area. One modality that has seemingly been accepted by most is that of telemedicine. NATO,adopted a standard definition of telemedicine as "the use of information and communications technologies to access healthcare regardless of time and distance."(5) It involves ready access to expert advice, medical knowledge and patient information in order to assist in the diagnosis, treatment, monitoring and management of patients. The deployment and utilization of telemedicine systems of varying complexities and for various purposes has been well-described elsewhere [1-4, 11, 12].

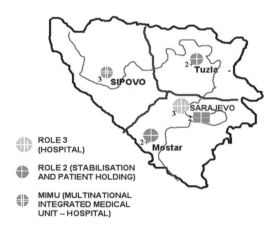

Figure 2. Medical Force Structure in Bosnia-Herzegovina (2000)

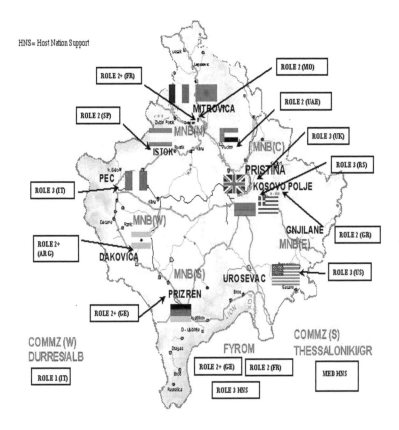

Figure 3. Medical Force Structure in Kosovo (2001)

2. NATO Telemedicine Organization

NATO has a well-developed standardization program that addresses many issues [6, 8, 9]. However, telemedicine interoperability telemedicine was not addressed until itlack became evident during operations in the Balkans. There NATO military medical forces could not effectively share digital medical information nor leverage information technology to coordinate medical care and evacuation. This has been complicated by the diverse array of information architectures and emerging proprietary national infrastructures for medical informatics, communications and telemedicine. The General Medical Working Group of

NATO (GMWG), recognizing that this issue needed resolution, invited presentations on the subject of Telemedicine in deployments at its June, 2000, meeting. After several presentations on topical issues, a two-day meeting of telemedicine experts from several nations was convened to develop a plan of action. After its initial meeting, this group recommended the development of Telemedicine standards and doctrine on a NATO-wide basis, and accordingly the GMWG established a permanent Telemedicine Panel to carry out the preliminary work.

The United States was chosen by the nations participating at the GMWG to provide the executive leadership for this group, and both the chairman and the secretary have been provided since its organization by personnel from the Office of the U.S. Army Surgeon General and the U.S. Army Telemedicine and Advanced Technology Research Center (TATRC) of the U.S. Army Medical Research and Materiel Command (USAMRMC).

The Telemedicine Panel is open to participation by all NATO members, as well as from all Partnership For Peace nations. Additionally, a representative from the Telemedicine Development Committee of the European Union has been invited to participate as an observer, to provide close links with similar efforts ongoing in the European Union civil sector. As of this writing, 18 nations participate in the work of the Panel, in addition to representatives of the European Union and various NATO commands.

Initial guidance given by the GMWG to the Panel included:

1. The U.S. will be the custodian for the development of a future telemedicine Standardization Agreement (STANAG), when such development is appropriate;
2. Before drafting a telemedicine STANAG, the Panel will develop an overarching policy statement for a NATO telemedicine STANAG and ensure review by the GMWG;
3. The Panel will develop new doctrinal policy for NATO on the subject of TMED operational development and utilization, and begin the staffing process to get this new policy ensconced in NATO doctrine;
4. As follow-on work, the Panel will identify discrete areas of a telemedicine STANAG which can be easily developed and adopted.

3. NATO Telemedicine Panel Focus

Beginning with few agreed notions as to what was either desirable or possible, the Panel decided on a staged approach. The overriding goal would be to collect and analyze prior telemedicine concepts developed from other organizations, rather than starting out to develop a concept for utilization "de novo". The effort was to first identify individual NATO member nations' concepts for deployable telemedicine systems, then to develop and promote a NATO "vision" for the use of telemedicine in providing medical care across the entire spectrum of potential military conflict. Rather than working in isolation, the Panel determined to leverage the telemedicine interoperability issues already being pursued by the NATO nations, the G-8 nations, various government telemedicine organizations, national telemedicine associations (technology special interest groups), industry, and the International Standards Organization (ISO).

Since its inception, the Telemedicine Panel has held nine meetings in various countries. Its Terms of Reference (NATO equivalent of Charter and Bylaws), have been approved, as well as significant progress toward the development of new NATO medical doctrine. To enable the Panel to focus clearly on an objective, Teleconsultation – a subcategory of telemedicine – was accepted as the primary focus of the Panel.

The goals of the operational medical structure in NATO with regard to telemedicine utilization during operations were identified early in the process, and the Allied Command Europe Medical Advisor's office of the Supreme Headquarters Allied Powers Europe (SHAPE) has been active in ensuring that developments meet the potential users' needs. As a result of this input, and discussion by the Panel members, a proposed requirement for Teleconsultation modalities at each given role/echelon (operational level) of care have been identified and approved by the Panel. (Figure 4)

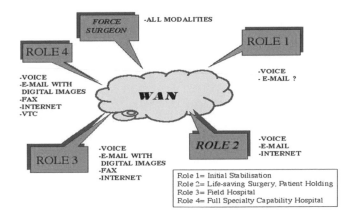

Figure 4. Proposed NATO Minimum Telemedicine Modality Requirements by Role

Throughout its series of meetings, the Panel has developed a proposed teleconsultation policy paper, setting forth its general recommendations for the development and use of telemedicine systems for teleconsultation during NATO operations.The policies and recommendations of this paper have been rewritten into a STANAG, which has been approved by the relevant NATO medical bodies, and is currently being staffed for ratification by the nations. When finally approved, this STANAG will form a part of NATO medical doctrine medical.

Key recommendations made by the Panel in this document include

1. Clinical operational concepts must be developed and validated before they are implemented or augmented with technical concepts;
2. Integration of telemedicine capabilities within military operations requires close attention to operational constraints;
3. Military telemedicine systems should be integrated within other strategic and tactical command, control, communications & intelligence systems;
4. Continuing and sustained training and integrated logistical support are essential;
5. Coalition military telemedicine operations require both technical and operational interoperability;
6. Store-and-forward teleconsultation has to date proven more useful for clinical care in field settings than has real-time video teleconferencing;
7. Development of a digital medical record would enhance the use and integration of telemedicine systems with other health services support; and
8. Telemedicine systems are used as much for situational awareness, medical command and control, and continuing medical education as for teleconsultation—these other uses are legitimate and their importance should not be underestimated.

Other efforts carried out by the Panel have included a review of all current NATO standardization and doctrine documents to determine their relevance to the operational deployment or use of telemedicine. A reference collection of these documents has been developed Panel and provided to its members and other interested bodies.

4. Telemedicine Panel Coordination

Early in the Panel's deliberations, it became obvious that these capabilities could not be developed in isolation. Hence, these capabilities must be fully integrated into the overall theater Medical Communications and Information Management Systems. Accordingly, investigation was carried out to determine an agency or body with responsibility in this area. The Committee of the Chiefs of the Military Medical Services in NATO (COMEDS) is the highest medical body within NATO, and is comprised of the Surgeons General of all the Alliance nations. It has numerous working groups involved in the development of medical doctrine and standards, one of which is the Medical Information Management Systems (MIMS) Working Group (WG).

5. TeleMED Interoperability Study

In examining the literature on operational telemedicine, it has become evident that there is a distinct lack of documentation about the clinical utility of various modalities of telemedicine in a multinational environment. Accordingly, the Panel has proposed a Telemedicine Interoperability Study (TiOPS) to be carried out in late 2004. This will involve the development by the researchers of a collection of telemedicine consultation packages (historical patient data sets). These packages will contain real patient conditions and documentation without individual indentification. Each package will include in digital format , basic relevant demographics (e.g. age, sex), a history of the present illness, a report of relevant physical and laboratory findings, and any useful illustrations, such as EKG, photographs, or X-Rays. Multiple nations will provide NATO Role 1-2 (forward medical facilities) to participate. These facilities will be provided with some of the patient data sets for test transmission via the Internet for consultation. These consultation requests will be sent to a secure web server operated by the researchers, which will serve as a consult router. This router will send each of the consults to several consultants from various nations, who will respond to the initiating facilities with their diagnoses, recommendations, and questions.   Thus, each initiating facility will receive multiple consultant responses to compare patient data.   To ensure full compatibility of systems, the same software for consultations, developed by the UK members of the Panel, will be provided to all participants. This will allow a determination of the "comfort" on the part of all participants with an international consult system; an evaluation of the usability at the initiating facility of any consultant responses; and an evaluation of the attitudes of consultants regarding the utility of the information.

6. Future Telemedicine Panel work

Current and proposed future work of the Panel includes:

1. Continued development of requirements for TMED systems which should be incorporated into the technical architecture being developed by the MIMS WG;
2. Continued development of the draft STANAG until it is incorporated into NATO medical doctrine and policy
3. Continued work on the development of teleconsultation standards and guidelines for use in a multinational environment
4. Carrying out and analyzing the proposed TiOPS study; and
5. Continuing to provide a forum for the exchange of lessons learned and problem solutions found in the fielding of national and multinational Telemedicine systems.

Acknowledgements

The authors wish to thank the members of the NATO TMED Panel, as well as Major General Lester Martinez-Lopez, Commander of the U.S. Army Medical Research and Materiel Command, and Colonel Jeffrey Roller, Director of the U.S. Army Telemedicine and Advanced Technology Research Center, for their continued strong support and encouragement for the work of the NATO Telemedicine Panel. Additionally, the support of the Charles McC. Mathias National Study Center for Trauma and Emergency Medical Systems, University of Maryland, Baltimore, Maryland and the Department of Electrical

Engineering, School of Engineering, University of Pittsburgh, Pittsburgh, Pennsylvania must be acknowledged. Without the time commitment permitted on the part of TATRC and University personnel, and the immense amounts of information provided to the Panel, we could not have accomplished as much as we have since our formation.

References

[1] Calcagni DE, Clyburn CA, Tomkins G, et al., Operation Joint Endeavor in Bosnia: telemedicine systems and case reports. Telemed J, 1996, 2,3:211-21.

[2] Clyburn CA, Gilbert GR, Cramer TJ, Lea RK, Ehnes SG, Zajtchuk R. Development of emerging telemedicine technologies with the Department of Defense: a case study of Operation Joint Endeavor in Bosnia. Acquisition Review Quarterly, 1997, 4, 1:101-121.

[3] Crowther, MAJ J. B. and LTC Ron Poropatich. Telemedicine in the U.S. Army: Case Reports from Somalia and Croatia, Telemed J , 1995, 1, 1:73-80.

[4] Gomez E, Poropatich R, Karinch MA, Zajtchuk J. Tertiary telemedicine support during global military humanitarian missions. Telemed J, 1996, 2, (3):201-210.

[5] NATO/COMEDS Telemedicine Panel, NATO Telemedicine Policy Paper and draft Teleconsultation STANAG, 2003.

[6] NATO Medical Staff Office. The NATO Medical Handbook. Brussels, Belgium: Headquarters NATO (IMS/LA&R Division), 2001.

[7] NATO Military Committee. MC 326/1-- NATO Medical Support Principles And Policies. Brussels, Belgium: Headquarters NATO, 1999.

[8] NATO Standardization Agency. AAP-3(H), Procedures For The Development, Preparation, Production And The Updating Of NATO Standardization Agreements (STANAGs) And Allied Publications (APs). Brussels, Belgium: Headquarters NATO, 2003.

[9] NATO Standardization Agency. AAP-4(2003), NATO Standardization Agreements) And Allied Publications). Brussels, Belgium: Headquarters NATO, 2003.

[10] NATO Standardization Agency. AJP 4.10, Allied Joint Medical Support Doctrine. Brussels, Belgium: Headquarters NATO, 2002.

[11] Navein J, Hagmann J, Ellis J. Telemedicine in support of peacekeeping operations overseas: an audit. Telemed J , 1997,3:207-214.

[12] Walters TJ. Deployment telemedicine: the Walter Reed Army Medical Center experience. Mil Med, 1996,161:531-536.

Redefining the Future of Healthcare Through Telecardiology and Telemedicine

Cristina RACOCEANU, George ILINCA

Infoworld, 37-39, Intrarea Glucozei Street, 2nd district, 023828, Bucharest, Romania

The paper was presented at the Advanced Research Workshop «Remote Cardiology Consultations Using Advanced Medical Technology – Applications for NATO Operations», held in Zagreb, Croatia 13-16 September 2005.

Developed by Info World, IQPACS is the first 100% Romanian ever built complete PACS, today implemented in Romania, Bulgaria and South Africa. The presentation shall be related to a special implementation of IQPACS called "The International Cardiology Network" using IQ Teleradiology, as well as call for new partners within healthcare institutions in this project.

With more than 7 years of expertise exclusively in the medical software field, more than 200 employees (140 involved in software development), being an Microsoft Gold Partner and ISO 9001:2001 certified, Info World is a supplier of IT solutions dedicated to the health field. We provide customized modular integrated solutions for both clinical and economic management of health care facilities. Info World also offers training, service and maintenance.

Info World is currently active in Europe, Latin America, Southern Africa and Asia, with more than 70 healthcare facilities using our solutions : hospitals, radiology centres, health insurance houses, laboratories, blood-banks, GP's, etc. and more than 3500 installed workstations. We have partnerships with C.A.C.I. (USA), ICT Works (South Africa), Fornax (Hungary), Alcatel, Fujitsu-Siemens and IBM.

Info World products (Hospital Manager Suite, Laboratory Manager, Budget Manager, Salary Manager, IQPACS, eFarma, Cabinet Manager, CTS Manager, CabiMed, ASIMED, eTest, Hippocrates, InFlow, ABC Net) create an integrated system customized for specific healthcare facilities, by also providing an integrated Electronic Health Record for each patient.

Since going international three years ago, Info World has developed projects and partnerships in more than 6 countries, as United States, Bulgaria, U.K., Columbia, Venezuela or South Africa.

Our strengths lie in having a proven / tested product base that define truly integrated solutions. We offer customizable solutions via a full service package with a reasonable pricing policy.

Our products are truly international, currently offered in Romanian, English, Spanish and Bulgarian (Cyrillic) and are based on the newest standards (like HL7, DICOM, etc).

New solutions and facilities developed by Info World (supporting e-Health and telemedicine):

- Nov. 2002 - Epinet / InFlow – on-line tool for automatic tracing and control of contagious diseases with-in a national system of data reporting
- Nov. 2003 – IQPACS includes module for Teleradiology
- Jan. 2004 – Hospital Manager Suite incorporates a new module, ABCnet, designed to offer secured on-line access both for patients and specialists to the Electronic Health Record kept in hospital database
- Sept. 2004 – HIMED becomes available – on-line tool for data reporting and exchange between hospitals, Public Safety Authority and Health Insurance House.
- Sept. 2004 – DesNet – National Electronic Health Record (part of National Trauma Network) – allows secure instant access to clinical record of any insured person when emergency occurs
- Oct 2004 – Hippo First Paperless practice management system Oct 2005 – Imhotep EMR - The core EMR allows physicians to enter history and physical information, notes, vital signs, etc. Allows for Physician Order Entry (POE) with Clinical Decision Support based on Knowledge based protocols

CASE STUDY: International Cardiology Network using IQ Teleradiology

- Info World started IQPACS implementation at "St. Ekaterina" Hospital in Sofia, immediately after finishing Hospital Manager HIS implementation there.
- "St. Ekaterina" Hospital in Sofia has an subsidiary in Odessa and longstanding contacts with The University Hospital in Graz, Austria, a hospital that has 1800 beds. It is part of The Styrian Hospital Organization, which manages 20 hospitals at 23 locations. All nine radiology institutes within the hospital group share an in-house RIS and a PACS.
- The three locations have different radiology resources, modalities and specialists.
- Two of our Romanian partners, "Heart Institute" from Cluj and "C.C. Iliescu" Cardiology Institute in Bucharest, became part of this project.

- The objective is to implement a solution that makes available sharing of resources in different locations in order to improve diagnosis and second opinion over a study, and usage of modalities without the need of patient or specialist to travel.
- The chosen solution was IQ Teleradiology module of IQPACS, both synchronous and asynchronous.
- Communication will be done through satellite connection, to ensure the best transmitting / receiving of studies and structured reports.

The following areas of cooperation are covered:

- Training and exchange programs between the hospitals, as the hospital in Graz has one of the largest and richest in technology and practice departments of image diagnostic
- "St. Ekatherina" has the first Multislice Spiral Computer tomography in Bulgaria but the hospital lacks experience in working with this modality
- The hospitals can obtain second opinion from each other
- Consultations about malformation and pathology
- Sharing greater experience
- Support specific groups of patients, which can be examined in one location but treated in another
- The project will be proposed for financing through European Union regional programmes; developing costs will be covered by Info World
- It is the first initiative in Cardiology, approaching an international network of specialists and modalities share-used
- The project is opened to new partners, both from public or private health sector
- It is currently under development.

Info World solutions:

- IQPACS Image Server
- IQPACS Diagnoses
- IQPACS Teleradiology

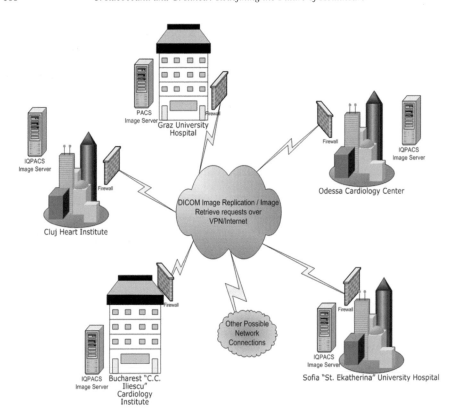

Remote Cardiology Consultations Using Advanced Medical Technology
I. Klapan and R. Poropatich (Eds.)
IOS Press, 2006

Telecardiological System for Acute Coronary Syndromes in Mazovia District of Poland

Robert RUDOWSKI[a] , Marcin GRABOWSKI[a,b] , Janusz SIERDZINSKI[a] , Filip SZYMANSKI[a,b]

[a] *Department of Medical Informatics and Telemedicine, Medical University of Warsaw*
SP CSK Hospital, Banacha Str. 1A, 02-097 Warsaw, Poland
[b] *Cardiology Clinic, I-st Faculty of Medicine, Medical University of Warsaw*

Abstract. Background: The high mortality in Poland due to the diseases of cardiovascular system (ca 50% of the total mortality) is the motivation for the presented work. Fight against those diseases is incorporated into e-health strategy for Poland for 2004-2006 and also into the National Program of Health. The interventional cardiology (angioplasty, sent implantation) combined with telecardiology can shorten the treatment delay and improve the outcomes of acute coronary syndrome (ACS) patients.

In Poland the interventional cardiology is performed only in big metropolitan centers to which the patients from smaller towns and rural areas need to be transported. Our system is addressed especially to those patients.

Aim: The aim of the work is the design and implementation of the prototype telecardiological system in Mazovia District (100 km radius around the capital Warsaw) with possible extension to other districts. Also improvement of cooperation among cardiological centers and rationalization of the specialized clinical resources and access to unified digital archives can be mentioned as the aims. The aim of medical importance is the reduction of time from symptoms to intervention which can possibly reduce mortality.

Methods: The overall structure of the system consists of 3 layers: 1 – reference (invasive cardiology) center, 2 – regional centers (hospitals), 3 – ambulance network. The software tools for communication among centers are Electronic Patient Record (EPR), accessible via Internet, relational data base MySQL in which EPR's are stored and expert system (ES) for risk assessment and advice on non-pharmacological treatment.

Result: EPR has been created up to now for over 100 patients. The data were stored in the database. ES performed risk stratification for each patient. It is based on the voting system in which risk scores such as SIMPLE, TIMI, GRACE, ZWOLLE are integrated with B-type natriuretic peptide (BNP). The patient is assigned to either low or high risk group which affects the choice of the type of treatment. ES evaluates also indications or contraindications for pharmacotherapy. Inter-rater agreement between a physician and ES was assessed by statistic kappa and was found either good (kappa 0,61-0,8) or very good (kappa 0,81-1).

Conclusion: The main elements of the system - EPR, database and ES are functioning properly. The regional centers require support in terms of staff training in EPR and database operation and also attention to the hardware, software and Internet access has to be paid for. Ambulance network is a crucial factor in improvement of healthcare of the ACS patients. Better cooperation among the regional and reference centers is required and also equipment for ECG data transmission over mobile phones.

The foreseen benefits of the system use are:
- better access to healthcare for the patients from rural areas and small towns,
- shortening the consultation time between ambulance/regional center and reference center which translates into shorter time from symptoms to intervention.

The paper was presented at the Advanced Research Workshop «Remote Cardiology Consultations Using Advanced Medical Technology – Applications for NATO Operations», held in Zagreb, Croatia 13-16 September 2005

1. Introduction

1.1 Cardiovascular Disease and Acute Coronary Syndromes in Poland

Cardiovascular Disease (CVD) including coronary heart disease causes nearly half of all deaths in Europe (49%) and in the EU (42%) and is the main cause of death in women and men in all countries of Europe. CVD is the main cause of years of life lost from early death in Europe and the EU – around one third of years of life lost from early death are due to CVD. CVD is the main cause of the disease burden (illness and death) in Europe (23% of all the disease burden) and the second main cause of the disease burden in the EU (18%). CVD is estimated to cost the EU economy €169 billion a year.

Coronary heart disease remains one of the main reasons of deaths and morbidity in Poland. It is nearly half of overall mortality (Fig. 1). However mortality due to CVD has continued to fall in Poland in both sexes and across educational levels. Compared with 1990, by 2002 for the age band 45-64 years it had fallen by 38% in men (340 per 100 000 to 212/100 000) and by 42% in women (76/100 000 to 44/100 000) [1]. Coronary heart disease leads to acute coronary syndrome (ACS) which is a life-threatening state. ACS are categorized, according to the presenting electrocardiogram (ECG) and results of necrotic markers, into non-ST-elevation myocardial infarction (non-STEMI), unstable angina (UA) and ST-elevation myocardial infarction (STEMI). Treatment is dependend on the category. Patients with non-STEMI/UA should be stabilized medically and scheduled for an early (within days) interventional strategy. Patients with STEMI should be treated acutely with thrombolysis or primary percutaneous coronary intervention (primary PCI), if admitted within 12 h of onset of symptoms [2,3].

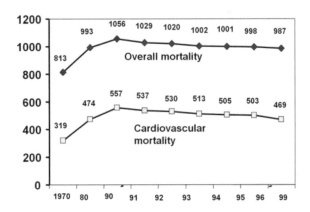

Figure 1. Overall and cardiovascular mortality in Poland between 1970 and 1999

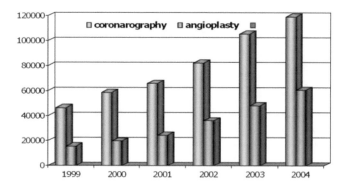

Figure 2. Coronarographies and angioplasties in Poland 1999-2004.

PCI offers benefits as compared to fibrinolysis for many patients with STEMI. This superiority of PCI in trials has led to the investigation of transfer strategies that would make PCI more widely available. Such a strategy would regionalize care and divert patients with STEMI to centers with PCI capability. The clinical cost of such a strategy in terms of time requires investigation [4].

To make a transfer strategy successful, it is essential to reduce the door-to-balloon time by improving systems and processes of care. To minimize the effect of the transfer on the time to reperfusion, communication should be optimized to include early mobilization of the cardiac catheterization laboratory team in the reference hospital. Efforts must be made to minimize delays on arrival at the hospital on the way to the catheterization laboratory. The randomized trials, as well as treatment networks now established in Poland, the Czech Republic, and isolated networks in the United States, demonstrate that this can indeed be accomplished [5].

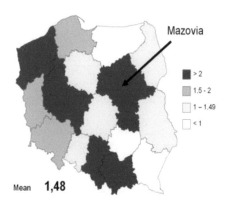

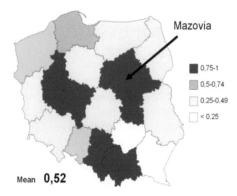

Figure 3. Accessibility of coronarographies in Poland per 1000 people in 2004.

Figure 4. Accessibility of angioplasties in Poland per 1000 people in 2004.

At this time in Poland we have 121 regular cardiology wards, 35 cardiology departments and 56 cardiology reference centers. Since the last five years in Poland the total number of coronarographies has been doubled (from 46 379 to 119 246) and the total number of angioplasties has increased 4 times (15 453 to 60 508) (Fig. 2). Mean ratio for 1000 people for coronarographies is 1,48 and for angioplasties is 0,52. Unfortunately there are districts in Poland with better accessibility of procedures and with worse accessibility (Fig. 3,4). At present there are 68 hospitals with cath lab and 51 of them work on 24 hours duty and are ready to treat immediately patients with ACS. Every year there are approximately 250 000 of ACS in Poland: 65% NSTEMI/UA and 35% STEMI. Nearly 40% of patients have been treated with PCI. In hospital mortality in centers with invasive procedures is 3-5 % but in hospitals without invasive treatment can be even 10-20%.

The number of patients with ACS treated with PCI in Poland still increases. But there is still a need for better selection of patients for early invasive strategy and for wider accessibility of invasive procedures for high risk patients. Telemedicine and telecommunication in terms of the ECG transmission from an ambulance to hospital or teleconsulations can be helpful and improve the situation.

1.2 Telecardiological System

Due to the development of telecommunication infrastructure some time ago a new direction appeared - telemedicine. The "radiomedicale" in Italy was precursor in this field. The medical services were provided for crews of ships at sea. The beginning of telemedicine in space was started with the flight of American astronaut John Glenn [6]. The electrical activity of his heart ECG was monitored. Due to the development of telecommunication and computer networks telemedicine settled in medical dictionary permanently and supports at present the protection of health.

Telemedicine comes from Greek word *"tele"* which means *"from a distance"* and Latin *"medicina"* which means *"medicine"* or *"medical art"* [7].

The key points to improve care of patients with ACS are:

- decreasing the time from the onset of symptoms to admission to hospital – patient decision
- decreasing the time of transport of patients from regional hospital to reference hospital cath lab
- initial risk stratification and selection of high risk patients from the whole group of patients with ACS – contact with physician from the reference hospital.

The project of telecardiological system was proposed to support the interventional cardiology in Mazovia District for ACS patients [8]. The system gathers systemized ACS patient data from the distant medical centers. It is expected to improve the co-operation among regional and reference medical centers. The next task of this system is to shorten the time from appearance of symptoms to undertaking treatment, what should reduce mortality.

The overall structure of the system consists of 3 layers (Fig. 5):

1 – reference (invasive cardiology) center, 2 – regional centers (hospitals), 3 – ambulance network. The software tools for communication among centers are Electronic Patient Record (EPR) accessible via Internet, relational data base MySQL in

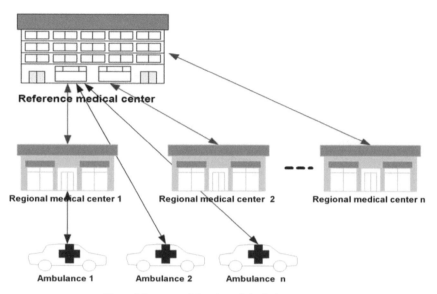

Figure 5. Structure of the telecardiological system.

which EPR's are stored and expert system (ES) for risk assessment and advice on non-pharmacological and pharmacological treatment.

2. Methods and Material

2.1. The concept of Electronic Patient Record (EPR)

The EPR is based on client-server architecture (Fig. 6).The EPR is implemented on a separate server, dedicated especially for operation under Linux system [9-10]. The Web server should have the PHP module to the database server (Apache). This means that the PHP tool is built into the WWW server, which helps to search the website. It is a combination of the programming language and the application server. For building EPR archives the relational database server MySQL was used. Its advantages are simplicity, high efficiency at low software requirements and speed of operation. It uses well known query language SQL. Several tools for creating EPR: PHP, HTML, XML and Java Script [11-16] were used.

EPR application has WWW interface. For operating it the acquaintance of Internet is sufficient. Doctor who is logging into the system is being authorized, and next from WWW site level he has access to data and results of patients' examinations from his own medical center. On this site a doctor has the possibility of filling the electronic forms with personal data and medical data. The history of the patient's disease is automatically generated. EPR application consists of several modules: Administrative, Registration and Login, Calls and Patients, Reports, Family Doctor as well as Attachments. The scheme of modules is shown in Fig 7.

EPR consists of the two main modules. The first one *Calls* is designed for fast transfer of medical data from regional centers to reference centers. Its main task is to support decision making related to patients who need help at once, which means

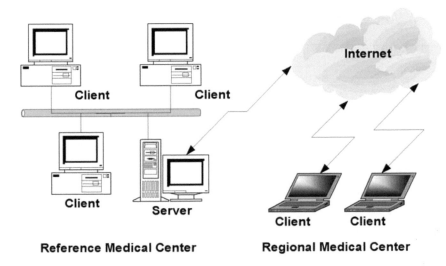

Figure 6. Structure of client-server EPR application in telecardiological system.

whether the patient is to be treated in a regional or reference center. This module contains a minimal number of forms to be sent to the data base. After performing these activities, SMS message is sent simultaneously to the physician on duty in the reference center. This physician has a duty to check the record of the patient which number has been sent to his phone. Decisions made according to the EPR will influence further procedures related to the patient.

The second module *Patients* is dedicated to physicians in regional centers as well as those in a reference center. Its main task is to collect detailed medical data about the patients. The work with two modules *Calls* and *Patients* is similar. In some forms there is a possibility of adding multiple new observations during one hospitalization (it applies only to forms in *Patients* module). Data from these forms are written down in the EPR data base. After filling the user can look through the whole record of the patient by clicking *Browse* link on the record page. The example of patient record is shown in Fig 8.

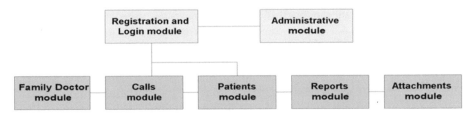

Figure 7. The modules of EPR.

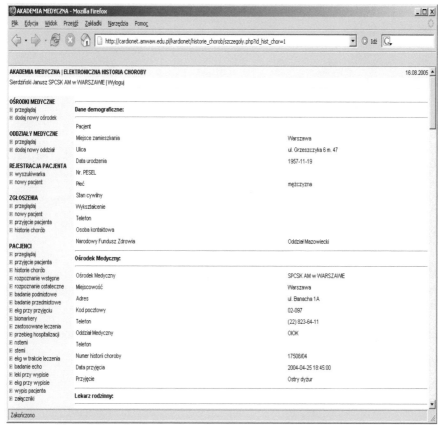

Figure 8.Example of electronic patient record in telecardiological system.

Apart from reviewing EPR the physician has the possibility to print it by clicking *Print* option. This option is accessible on every page of application, which facilitates printing the forms as well as getting familiar with them. The module of adding the files of different formats is implemented in several forms (eg. ECG).

In menu, different modules are visible such as: *Reports, Family Doctor and Attachments*.

Reports module is designed to report the daily history of events for every patient. *Family Doctor* allows for addition of new family doctors to the system.

The module *Attachments* is connected with adding the ECG files to the database. We can use it both from menu panel and directly from forms.

Due to easy presentation of data in a formalized form with the usage of XML (*Extensible Markup Language*), as well as its perfect cooperation with databases – it has a very important meaning in EPR. XML file, apart from possibility of displaying it in Internet browser, is a starting point for introducing the communication standard of medical textual data HL7 [7-18].

2.2. Database Architecture

The database is a relational database. The basic property of such database is that the data is stored in tables with defined relations among them. All tables in **am_ehc** are

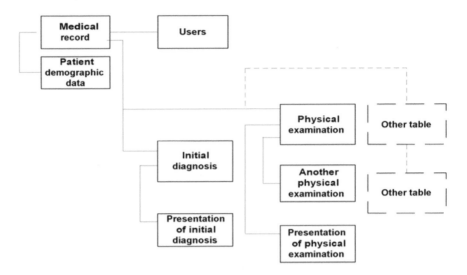

Figure 9.The scheme of EPR relational database

designed in such a way that there is no redundant information [11-16,19] (Fig. 9). Tables are used for collection and storage of data from medical questionnaires and are divided in 3 groups:
- for data storage
- for data presentation
- for identifiers defining the possibility of entering the data once again from medical questionnaires.

2.3. System administration and data security

A global administrator main task is to take care of the server with regard to software timeliness. Proper configuration and error free software make the server safe and secure. Standard administrator tasks, including creating backups, changes in system configuration etc., establish the foundation of the internet site secure system.

The main place to execute administrator activities in the Electronic Patient Record is the administrative panel. It is a place where operations like conferring authorizations upon using the EPR database, removing user accounts, which are no longer using the system, removing old and useless files or incomplete medical records are carried out. These activities are accessible only for appointed persons from a given center, who are local administrators as shown in Fig 10. Another part of database administration is conferring authorizations upon users working with EPR system. These authorizations were divided into groups with regard to the type of the user. Possibility of removing patients' medical records is reserved only to the user called administrator. Next two groups: resident and physician personnel have the rights to add, edit and review only these patients' medical records, whose data they introduced. The last group-guests, is created for students and third persons who may only review anonymous patients' records without rights to modify them.

Burglaries to internet servers are nothing extraordinary. In order to counteract them, firewalls and detection systems are being used. Yet, these operations cannot completely eliminate the risk. We should start with the aspect of data transmission security.

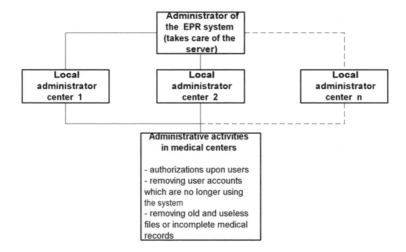

Figure 10. The scheme of administrative activities

TCP/IP protocol doesn't have own encrypting functions build-in. Also HTTP based on from TCP/IP, doesn't assure data security. All data are sent in a transparent way and are exposed to be investigated and intercepted. Different cryptographic methods are being used to prevent these situations. HTTPS is an extended version of the HTTP for encrypting the data sent between clients and server. HTTPS ensures secure connection and is actually implemented in all modern www browsers. Also EPR application is using this protocol. During the HTTPS connection data is encrypted with the usage of the key generated with help of SSL library. The data becomes unreadable and because of this, useless to unauthorized persons (9-16, 19).

A very important question, concerning security, is code hiding. If a potential hacker doesn't know what script is doing, what the architecture of our database is, he can only guess. In EPR application login and password to the database is not accessible from the www server level. Moreover, password is collected from the form by using password option, which assures its hiding. In EPR application, use of global variables is avoided. In this way we are secure from the hacker interference by initiating database variables via URL address.

Another security feature used in EPR is a session investigation method. This method not so much transfers parameters but rather stores little quantity data in a site visitor's computer (i.e. by generating this visit identifier). Next transitions from site to site may transfer it. If there will be no identifier, the site we want to review would not be shown again.

The range of the administrative activities in EPR database and the data security is mostly based on the confidence of all persons who may approach it. Physicians and medical personnel work should be based on limited confidence degree regarding third persons, who may influence data and the whole system security.

2.4. Expert System

The expert system supporting risk stratification and early treatment in acute coronary syndromes was developed and was integrated with the database. Knowledge base contains rules according to the current guidelines of the European Society of

Cardiology [2]. Expert system consists of: a) risk voting system which votes on risk on the basis of points counted according to 4 risk scores (SIMPLE, TIMI STEMI, GRACE, ZWOLLE) and on BNP (Fig. 11); b) module suggesting the type of reperfusion therapy (invasive vs. fibrynolisis); c) module which chooses pharmacotherapy. Inter rater agreement between the expert system and the physician-expert was determined by kappa statistic.

2.5. Risk Stratification

Management of ACS should be guided by an estimate of patient risk. Risk stratification in ACS aims at prompt identification of the higher-risk patient who will profit from aggressive investigation and therapy and of the lower-risk patient who can advantageously be treated more conservatively. Risk stratification is based on patient history, physical examination, electrocardiogram and biochemical markers. There are some new markers, such as B-type natriuretic peptide (BNP) with proven prognostic power.

An emerging approach to ACS is to use a comprehensive approach to risk assessment. Risk scores (eg. SIMPLE, TIMI STEMI, GRACE, ZWOLLE) were developed to facilitate early risk stratification. They incorporate important demographic, clinical, ECG and blood marker parameters shown to be independent predictors of prognosis in multiple regression analyses of different databases. Risk stratification with scoring system on admission offers the best way to identify high risk patients who would benefit most from invasive treatment. Clinical predictors can be included in computer programs such as expert systems and used in risk stratification. This can be helpful in decision making for ACS patients [20,21].

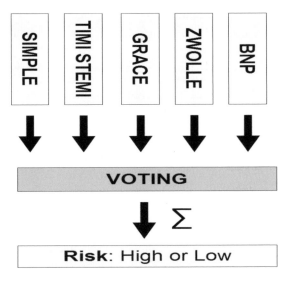

Figure 11. Risk voting system which votes on risk on the basis of points counted according to 4 risk scores (SIMPLE, TIMI STEMI, GRACE, ZWOLLE).

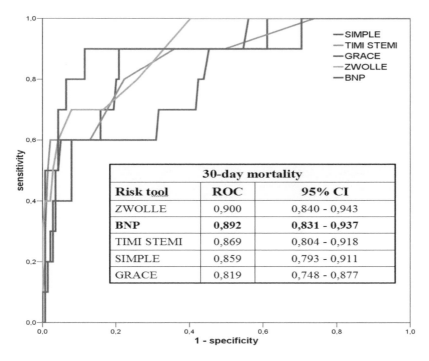

Figure 12. Areas under ROC curves for risk scores and BNP.

2.6. Material

The system was evaluated on medical data of 149 consecutive patients hospitalized due to ACS. Patients were transferred from regional hospitals or came on their own to Admission Department of University Hospital. All patients were admitted to Cardiology Clinic. Clinical data, ie history, risk factors, physical examination, electrocardiogram, laboratory results, were analyzed by qualified physicians. All data were put into EPR and into the expert system. Risk stratification was done. After that patients were sent to cath lab and PCI was performed. After discharge continuous follow-up of patients was performed, by now most patients finished 2 year follow-up.

3. Results

Baseline BNP levels were higher among patients who died compared to those who survived first 30 days (mean: 652,09 vs. 144,4 pg/ml, p<0,0001). BNP showed strong predicting value for 30-day mortality – area under ROC curve was 0,892 (95% confidence interval [CI]: 0,831 - 0,937). BNP at level of 334 pg/ml had 90,0% sensitivity (95%CI: 55,5- 98,3) and 88,5% specificity (95%CI: 82,0- 93,3) for prediction of 30-day mortality. In multivariate analysis BNP levels were independent risk factor of death at 30-days (odds ratio=40,6, 95%CI 4,5 – 370,1, p<0,001). Areas under ROC curves for risk scores were for: SIMPLE - 0,859 (95%CI: 0,793 - 0,911), TIMI STEMI - 0,869 (95%CI: 0,804 - 0,918), GRACE - 0,819 (95%CI: 0,748 - 0,877), ZWOLLE - 0,9 (95%CI: 0,84 - 0,943) (Fig. 13). There was no good agreement

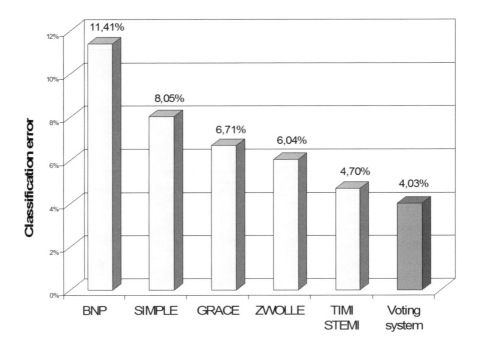

Figure 13. Classification error for risk scores and BNP.

between BNP levels and risk scores in risk stratification. In multivariate analysis incorporating BNP and each risk score separately, BNP remained independent risk factor for 30-day mortality. The addition of BNP into the model increased ROC. Classification error for risk scores and BNP were: for SIMPLE - 8,05%; TIMI STEMI - 4,70%; GRACE - 6,71%; ZWOLLE - 6,04%; BNP - 11,41% (Fig. 13). Developed majority voting system had the lowest classification error - 4,03%. The additional calculations for voting system with different cut-off points for high risk have been performed. The best sensitivity was obtained in system with 1 vote needed for high risk assessment: sensitivity 90%, specificity - 84,2%, classification error- 15,44%. The best specificity was obtained in system with 4 votes needed for high risk assessment: sensitivity 30%, specificity - 100%, classification error- 4,7%. Our strategy is that high sensitivity is required in regional hospitals not to overlook high risk patients. High specificity is needed in reference hospitals. All patients there are treated with PCI but very high risk patients should receive additional treatment procedures. Full agreement was seen between physician-expert and expert system in decision for the need of reperfusion therapy; good agreement in decision for the type of reperfusion therapy (kappa=0,65), good for angiotensin converting enzyme inhibitors (kappa=0,69), beta-adrenolitics (kappa=0,705), nitroglycerin (kappa=0,69), furosemide (kappa=0,72), very good agreement for aspirin (kappa=0,889) and full (kappa =1) for heparin (Fig. 14).

4. Discussion

The electronic patient record has been created for patients from SP CSK AM Hospital (reference center) and for patients from the regional centers remotely. Clinical data were put into EPR by staff from both kinds of centers. This confirmed system operation and verified applied solutions. EPR is used for patients' data collection. Reports can be printed and attached to paper record. Patients are followed up. Collected data gives overview of patients profile and allows to make analyzes of treatment efficacy. Unfortunately, paper patient record has to be generated in parallel to EPR. Our final aim is to replace traditional paper record with developed EPR. For that purpose computer equipment and network will be needed at all points of Cardiology Clinic and in associated labs eg. biochemistry, radiology etc. Full training of staff also will have to be done.

Data from patients were analyzed by developed expert system which performed risk stratification and suggested treatment. Good and very good agreement was observed between expert system and physician-expert in type of therapy (reperfusion, pharmacotherapy) choice. Addition of a new biochemical marker - BNP - into popular risk scores improved risk stratification in patients with ACS. Developed voting system significantly decreased classification error to risk groups. Changes in cut-off for votes on high risk improved sensitivity or specificity for risk classification dependently on the reference level of cardiological center.

At this stage the system is ready to use. Unfortunately there are some barriers which make implementation difficult. Firstly, some regional centers have problems with access to internet and with computer equipment mainly due to small financial resources. The second problem is lack of equipment which allows ambulances to transmit electrocardiogram to reference hospitals. Thirdly, there is a need to develop better cooperation among reference hospitals in Mazovia District. At this time the information on free monitored beds in reference hospitals is very uncertain. Finally, present law in Poland does not allow full implemtation of EPR.

Summarizing, great effort has been made to develop presented system which has been positively evaluated in practice. Now there is a need for wider implementation which requires cooperation among hospitals, some logistic solutions and decisions made by local authorities and heads of hospitals and departments, and last but not least financial resources.

The project of presented telecardiological system supports "e-health" strategy for Poland 2004-2006 and the National Program of Health. Both initiatives mention the fight against coronary diseases as one of their strategic aims.

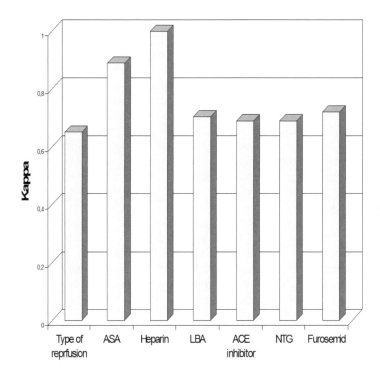

Figure 14. Agreement between physician-expert and expert system – results of kappa statistic.

References

[1]   Zatonski WA. Changes in dietary fat and declining coronary heart disease in Poland: population based study. BMJ 2005; 331: 187–188.
[2]   Van de Werf F, Ardissino D, Betriu A, Cokkinos DV, Falk E, Fox KA, Julian D, Lengyel M, Neumann FJ, Ruzyllo W, Thygesen C, Underwood SR, Vahanian A, Verheugt FW, Wijns W. Management of acute myocardial infarction in patients presenting with ST-segment elevation. Eur Heart J 2003;24:28–66.
[3]   Braunwald E, Antman EM, Beasley JW, Califf RM, Cheitlin MD, Hochman JS, Jones RH, Kereiakes D, Kupersmith J, Levin TN, Pepine CJ, Schaeffer JW, Smith EE 3rd, Steward DE, Theroux P, Gibbons RJ, Alpert JS, Faxon DP, Fuster V, Gregoratos G, Hiratzka LF, Jacobs AK, Smith SC Jr. ACC/AHA guideline update for the management of patients with unstable angina and non-ST-segment elevation myocardial infarction—2002: summary article: a report of the American College of Cardiology/American Heart Association Task Force on Practice Guidelines (Committee on the Management of Patients with Unstable Angina). Circulation 2002;106:1893–1900.
[4]   Keeley EC, Boura JA, Grines CL. Primary angioplasty versus intravenous thrombolytic therapy for acute myocardial infarction: a quantitative review of 23 randomized trials. Lancet. 2003;361:13–20.
[5]   Herrmann HC, Transfer for Primary Angioplasty. The Importance of Time. Circulation. 2005;111:718-720.

[6]   Beolchi L, (Ed.). European Telemedicine Glossary of Concepts, Standards, Technologies and Users. European Commision, 2001.

[7]   Duplaga M. Telemedicine and e-health as consecutive stages of development of telemedical systems in health care (in Polish). Zdrowie i Zarządzanie, 2003; vol. V, 1.

[8]   Opolski G, Filipiak K J, Poloński L etel., (Eds.). Acute Coronary Syndromes (in Polish), Urban & Partner, Wrocław, 2002:1-11.

[9]   Butzen F, Forbes B. Linux Data Base. Warszawa, 1999.

[10] Kirch O, Dawson T. Linux Network Administrator's Guide. O'Reilly & Associates, 2000.

[11] Valade J. PHP 5 For Dummies, Wiley Publishing, Inc, Indianapolis, Indiana, 2004.

[12] Converse T, Park J, Morgan C. PHP5 and MySQL Bible, Wiley Publishing, Inc, Indianapolis, Indiana, 2004.

[13] Rockwell W. XML, XSLT, Java, and JSP: A Case Study in Developing a Web Application, Galileo Press GmbH Bonn, Germany, 2000.

[14] Vaswani V. XML and PHP, New Riders Publishing, 2002.

[15] Harold E R. XML.Expert Book (in Polish), Helion, Gliwice, 2000.
[16] Hugh E W, Lane D. Web Database Applications with PHP & MySQL, O'Reilly & Associates, Inc, 2002.
[17] Heitmann K. The German SCIPHOX project, Int. Conf. on the HL7 Clinical Document Architecture (CDA). Berlin (Germany), 7-9.10.2002:13.

[18] Heitmann KU, Schweiger R, Dudeck J. Discharge and referral data exchange using global standards – The SCIPHOX project in Germany. Medical Informatics Europe, IOS Press, 2002:679-684.

[19] Rudowski R. etel., (Ed.). Medical Informatics (in Polish), PWN, Warszawa, 2003.

[20] Grabowski M, Filipiak KJ, Karpinski G, Wretowski D, Rdzanek A, Huczek Z, Horszczaruk GJ, Kochman J, Rudowski R, Opolski G. Serum B-type natriuretic peptide levels on admission predict not only short-term mortality but also angiographic success of procedure in patients with acute ST elevation myocardial infarction treated with primary angioplasty. American Heart Journal 2004;148:655–662.
[21] Grabowski M, Filipiak KJ, Rudowski R, Opolski G. Project of an expert system supporting risk stratification and therapeutic decision making in acute coronary syndromes. Polish Journal of Pathology 2003;54:205-208.

Development of Diagnostic Cardiology/Telecardiology Procedures in Republic of Moldova

Adela STAMATI[a], Mihail POPIVICI[b]

[a] Departement of pediatric cardiology, State Medical and Pharmaceutical University "Nicolae Testemitanu"; scientific secretary at Experts Council, Minister of Health and Social Protection of Republic of Moldova
[b] Director of Institute of Cardiology, Republic of Moldova

Abstract. Cardiovascular disease (CVD) has emerged as the dominant chronic disease in many parts of the word. At the beginning of the 21st century, CVD account for nearly half of all deaths in the developed world and about twenty five percent in the developing word. Cardiological Service in Republic of Moldova is a structure relatively young and it is in permanent reshape. There are no national data on the real number of cardiac patients. Epidemiological studies of terrain (1998-2002) have shown that there are enormous differences of usage of new technologies in different regions. We have big problems with insufficient financing of health and public cardiological service. The future national Program of prevention and treatment of CVD will have the aim to contribute to find out all of cardiac patients and distinguish the groups of high risk from the healthy population. Based on the epidemiological situation we need to elaboration some national project, including as e-health, Telemedicine/Telecardiology for implementation in our health system.

The paper was presented at the Advanced Research Workshop «Remote Cardiology Consultations Using Advanced Medical Technology – Applications for NATO Operations», held in Zagreb, Croatia 13-16 September 2005

1. Introduction

At the beginning of the third millennium, national health and diseases profiles very change by geographical region and by country. The technological progress and their associated economic and social transformations have resulted in dramatic shifts in structure of human diseases and death.

A thus cardiovascular disease (CVD) has emerged as the dominant chronic disease in many parts of the word. At the beginning of the 21st century, CVD account for nearly half of all deaths in the developed world and about twenty five percent in the developing word.[1,2] Sudden cardiac death in the young (≤ 35years) has a structural basis in up to 80% of cases. [3,4]

Our country is in a period of transition to a better democracy and a stronger economy. Economical crises from 1994 (nineteen hundred ninety four) have not past yet in totally in our Republic. It influenced negatively all social and economical departments including the one responsible of Public Health. Our slow economy progress has impoverished the population which beneficiated health assistance from government's budget. Some of those experiences are it is implemented the Family Medicine (more 5 years of activity), obligatory Health Insurance (2 years activity), elaboration and implement of medical standards diagnosis and treatment by medical specialization, it is working on elaboration of guides and protocols. I say all these things to mention that in countries like Moldova it is almost impossible to make the necessary modern reshape in public health system without international help and collaboration.

We want to mention that Cardiological Service in Republic of Moldova is a structure relatively young and it is in permanent reshape. There are no national data on the real number of cardiac patients.

2. Materials and Methods

Epidemiological studies of terrain (1998-2002) have shown that there are enormous differences of usage of new technologies in different regions. We have big problems with insufficient financing of health and public cardiological service. The principals of new technologies have been applied prevalent in the Institute of Cardiology from our capital, Chisinau. The future national Program of prevention and treatment of CVD will have the aim to contribute to find out all of cardiac patients and distinguish the groups of high risk from the healthy population. Based on the epidemiological situation we need to elaboration some national project, including as e-health, Telemedicine/Telecardiology for implementation in our health system.

3. Results

The majority of population of Republic of Moldova is a rural one (58.6% (fifty eight point six percent) out of 4 millions). The rural population is the most vulnerable in our country that is why at this population health indexes got worse.

Table 1. Demographical structure of population from Republic of Moldova (without Transnistria)

Estimated categories	Measures	1995	1996	1997	1998	1999	2000	2001	2002
Total population	Thousands of people	3604	3599	3654	3652	3646	3635,1	3627,8	3617,7
Men Women	%	47,8 52,2	47,8 52,2	47,8 52,2	47,8 52,2	47,8 52,2	47,9 52,1	47,9 52,1	- -
Urban area Rural area	%	42,8 57,2	42,8 57,2	42,2 57,8	42 58	42 58	40,9 59,1	40,9 59,1	41,4 58,6
Density	People/km^2	128,6	128,2	127,8	127,4	127	127	126	126

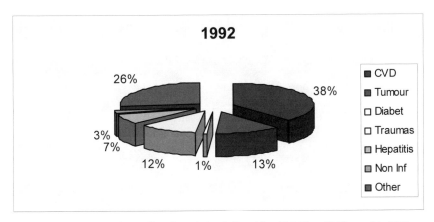

Figure 1. Structure of mortality of population in Republic of Moldova (0-99 years) in 1992

In this table is presented social and demographical situation in our country without Transnistria during 10 years where prevalent are women and population density remains high in spite of the increase of migration.

For countries like Republic of Moldova and other East-European countries it is typical the demographical tendencies like:
-    The decrease of the number of population able to work (16-60 years)
-    The decrease of natality
-    The increase of mortality caused by non infectious diseases

All Health indexes show the public health was affected by economical situation.

In the structure of mortality causes of population in our country we observe that in 2002 (two thousands two) prevails cardiovascular diseases (56.7% fifty six point seven percent) and the most frequent are ischemic disease and the stroke. At population able to work the cardiovascular disease is very high, too.

Official statistics shows that the mortality increased considerable because of cardiovascular diseases among the population of Republic of Moldova in the last 10 years (from 38% thirty eight percent in 1992 to 56% fifty six percent in 2002 (Figures 1,2).

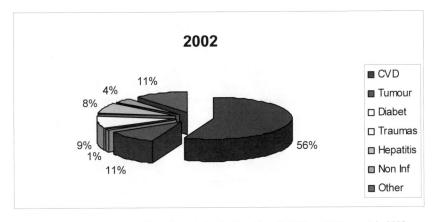

Figure2. Structure of mortality of population in Republic of Moldova (0-99 years) in 2002.

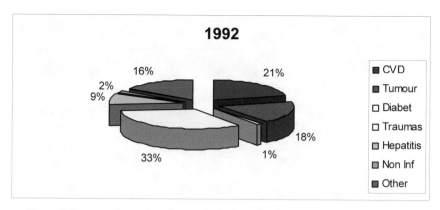

Figure 3. Structure of mortality of population in Republic of Moldova (16-60 years) in 1992.

The same increase we have at young population too (from 21% percent in 1992 to 24% twenty two percent in 2002). (Figure 3,4).

Cardiovascular mortality influences the span of life in Moldova. In the last it is observed a tendency of increase of span of life similar to year 1992. (Figure 5)

Epidemiological studies of terrain and local ones showed us because of this problems 62% of population that are ill will the risk of cardiovascular diseases are not traced out in time. Over 30% of adult populations don't know their arterial pressure, body weight, glycemic level and other health indexes. At the same time in that period the number of specialists in cardiology has reduced, so the statistics of the end of 2002 year is: 1 cardiologist / 100 000 (one hundred thousands) people and 1 cardiologic bed/ 400 (four hundreds) people.

The future National Program of Prevention and Treatment of Cardiovascular Diseases will have the aim to contribute to the decrease of mortality and morbidity caused by cardiovascular diseases and by increasing the quality life of cardiac patients. Using present recommendation of the European Society of Cardiology and World Health Organization, other our task is to implement new technologies of diagnosis and treatment. The main objective is that in a short period (till 5 years) is the subtraction of the absolute risk of coronary disease and other arteriopathies of atherosclerotic etiology (central and peripherical). The objective of the long period (5-10 years) is the reduction of cardiac morbidity and mortality of atherosclerotic etiology, the increase of hope life and its quality.

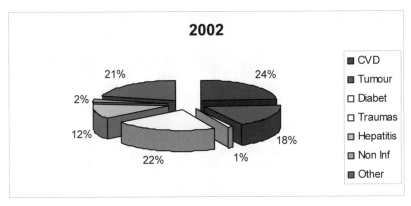

Figure 4. Structure of mortality of population in Republic of Moldova (16-60 years) in 2002.

4. Discussion

Telemedicine is only at the beginning in our country but my colleagues from different specialties work hard to introduce the basis of telemedicine. There is a project that works now at State Medical and Pharmaceutical University "Nicolae Testemitanu" and my colleagues give consultations on phone and it is not only in Chisinau our capitol but in Balti – northern capitol.

Government's decision dated on 14th October 2004 was the basis of introduction of new state informational system. It is called: "Regarding the approval of the Conception of medical integrated informational system."

The possibility to realize this decree came true in March 2005, when a new governmental Ministry was inaugurated: The Ministry of Informational Development of Republic of Moldova.

On 7th July 2005 took place the first meeting of the Ministry of Informational Development with the Ministry of Health and Social Protection - "round table". During the meeting it was established the current stage of creation in informational society of e-Health.

The project of development of Telemedicine system includes some next prerogatives:
-   To endow medical institutions with computers and all necessary technical equipments.
-   To elaborate and to implement the pilot-projects on specialties (Hancesti).
-   To create the Service System of Telemedicine.
-   To create the program of education at distance for specialists from Health care etc.

But Telecardiology is not active in our country yet.

Our common problems are: technical insurance – it is not modern and it is insufficient, and our population has not enough knowledge about foreign languages like English. We are in this situation because Moldova is a young country. It exists as separated independent country only for 14 years so our democracy can not be compared with the one in Western Europe and USA. In time step by step Moldova will overcome its problems and it will have a place near other democratic countries. We have well prepared specialists in cardiology and management who want to promote Telemedicine/telecardiology in Republic of Moldova, but we have much to learn from experiences of other developed countries. [5]

References

[1]   Sans S, Kesteloot H, Kromhout D. The burden of cardiovascular diseases mortality in Europe. Task Force of the European Society of Cardiology on Cardiovascular Mortality and Morbidity Statistics in Europe. Eur Heart J, 1997, 18: 1231-48.
[2]   Murray CJL, Lopez AD. The Global Burden of Disease. Cambridge, MA, Harvard School of Public Health, 1996.
[3]   Bowker TJ, Wood DA, Davies MJ, et al. Sudden unexpected cardiac or unexplained death in England: a national survey. QJM, 2003, 96: 269-279.
[4]   Semsarian C, Maron BJ. Sudden cardiac death in the young. Med J Aust, 2002, 176: 148-149.
[5]   Klapan I., Čikeš I. Telemedicine. Zagreb; Telemedicine Association, 2005.

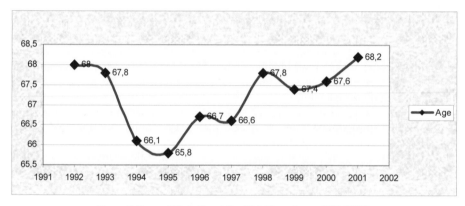

Figure 5. Span of life in Republic of Moldova (years 1991-2002).

Croatia and NATO

Aleksandar SUNKO
Department for NATO, Political, Military and Security Issues
Republic of Croatia, Ministry of foreign affairs, 1st political division for the European
Union, NATO and member countries

The paper was presented at the Advanced Research Workshop «Remote Cardiology Consultations Using Advanced Medical Technology – Applications for NATO Operations», held in Zagreb, Croatia 13-16 September 2005

1. Introduction

The purpose of this presentation is to outline in brief, how international co-operation in medicine fits into the wider picture of Croatia – NATO relations.

Apart from being a European Union candidate country (the European Union Council of Ministers decided, on October 4, 2005, to open accession negotiations with Croatia), Croatia is embarking on its fourth cycle of the Membership Action Plan which is designed to help Croatian membership to NATO.

Croatia values Euro-Atlantic integration as the priority of its foreign policy. Croatia views its membership in NATO and the EU as the best guarantee of its security and prosperity. It's not just that Croatia, as a modern democratic society, belongs to the European Family, but its strong Euro-Atlantic commitment is founded both culturally and historically. Croatia wishes to make a most effective contribution to the community of European and Euro-Atlantic democracies whose common foundations it shares, while taking up fully its responsibilities.

The new ANP (Annual National Plan) has been presented at the NATO Headquarters in Bruxelles in October 2005. As stated in the Plan, within the scope of the current defence reform, the aim is, inter alia, that of creating a modern and efficient military force in Croatia, capable of handling global and asymmetric challenges, depending on NATO membership and security arrangements in the EU framework. The emphasis of the reforms taking place is on the development of capabilities for participation in Allied operations. Forces that are being developed are to be fully professional, mobile, deployable and financially affordable.

2. International defense co-operation

International defense co-operation is an important instrument of capabilities enlargement and interoperability of Croatia's military forces (most intense bilateral cooperation is with the following states: USA, Great Britain, Germany, France, Austria, Italy, Hungary and Slovenia; a total of 581 activities in the time span of 2 ANP cycles). Croatia's future membership in NATO will have a positive influence on the long term stabilization process of South East Europe through the expansion of the areas of stability, security and through the acceptance of common values and economic prosperity. It is important to emphasize that Croatia's regional neighbors fully support Croatia's Euro-Atlantic ambitions.

Continued development of good relations with neighbouring countries is a priority. With the neighbouring Member States of NATO and the EU a close cooperation is under way, aimed at utilising and learning from their integration experiences. Croatia supports the EU and NATO aspirations of Bosnia-Herzegovina and Serbia and Montenegro

The value of regional co-operation as a part of Croatian foreign and defence policy is paramount, given its contribution to regional security and stability in Europe. This co-operation also stems from the obligations and criteria set for Croatia in the process of NATO-integration. It has proven valuable in the framework of Croatian participation in international operations. In this context, the so-called U.S.-Adriatic charter is a useful instrument. Within the format of the U.S.-Adriatic Charter of Partnership, Croatia co-operates with two other NATO aspirants, Albania and Macedonia, and with the U.S., on projects which have concrete, well defined goals. As discussed bellow, the fruitfulness of this co-operation is demonstrated by the assignment of a combined trilateral military medical team to Afghanistan.

3. Afghanistan

It is of great importance to note the Croatian contribution to the ISAF NATO Mission in Afghanistan. Its importance lies also in the context of international co-operation in medicine. With the ambition of furthering its efforts in ISAF, Croatia, together with other two US-Adriatic Charter countries, set up a joint military medical team for ISAF, 11 persons strong, deployed in August. It is supporting medical care on KAIA – Kabul Afghanistan International Airport Yet again, establishing fully functioning and developed "telemedicine" will provide immense help in the ground work of our military medical team in Afghanistan. In the so-called Provincial Reconstruction Team (PRT) in the Afghan Province of Feyzabad (in the North-East of the country), a Croatian Diplomat is the Deputy Director of Civilian Affairs. In the same mission, under German leadership, Croatia also participates with its police officers. The professional performance of the Croatian contingent in the ISAF mission has been widely praised by the Commander of ISAF (COMISAF) and other local and international actors in Afghanistan.

4. Iraq and Other Missions

In a period of five years Croatia has gone from a user to an important participant of peacekeeping missions, taking part in missions around the world. Apart from Afghanistan, Croatia is momentarily participating in the following UN peacekeeping missions: Sierra Leone, Eritreia-Ethiopia, India/Pakistan, Ivory Coast, Liberia, Western Sahara, Cyprus ad Haiti. Preparations are being done for future participation in Georgia, Lebanon and the Golan Plains. Croatia participated in Bosnia's SFOR mission and Kosovo's KFOR, and is completely supporting EU's new mission *Althea* which is to become functional by the end of the year. In the field of civil police support, Croatia has sent its first 3-man instructor team to the International police academy in Jordan, in

June 2005, where Iraqi police officers are being trained. Possibilities of providing training and education for Iraqi Armed Forces in Croatia are to be explored.

Away from direct engagement in crisis areas, and as a part of humanitarian aid to the population of Iraq, in the second half of 2004, Croatia received seven seriously ill Iraqi children, aged 2 to 11, for treatment in Croatian hospitals. After successful treatment all of the children returned to their country. At the same time, six Iraqi physicians attended forensic courses in Croatia. In the following cycle it is specifically intended to continue co-operation in the area of providing training for the Iraqi staff in forensic medicine as a part of the project aimed at establishing a system of victim identification by means of DNA analysis. This is another example of the emphasis Croatia places on its medical expertise, as part of the country's activities in assisting international peace keeping and humanitarian operations. It is worth noting in this context, that the Croatian Navy has a Maritime Medicine Institute within its structure.

5. Weapons of Mass Destruction, Terrorism, Organised Crime and Trafficking

Participation will be intensified in a number of other activities against international terrorism and the proliferation of weapons of mass destruction. Special attention will be paid to improving border security, aimed at waging an efficient fight against terrorism, smuggling, organised crime and human trafficking. In co-operation with the OSCE, the Croatian National Committee against the Human Trafficking organised several events on the subject, with the intention of raising public awareness concerning this problem, and its various aspects – political, legal, social, and medical.

Croatia has acceded or is in the process of acceding to all relevant international mechanisms on countering the weapons of mass destruction proliferation. Recently, in September 2005, Croatia hosted a workshop on Chemical, Biological and Radiological Terrorism. Scientific research and medical know-how are thus clearly demonstrated going hand in hand with Croatia-NATO co-operation.

6. Conclusion

All of these activities, and peace missions abroad in particular, have great importance not just as an expression of Croatian readiness to fully join NATO Alliance as equal member but as an expression of how a small country can actively contribute to efforts around the world aiming at enhancing peace, stability, security and human well-being. In conjunction with purely political, security and military ramifications that these efforts may have, close co-operation with the scientific and medical community is a self-evident necessity. The title of the NATO programme covering this Advanced Research Workshop, is *Security through Science*. This is a highly appropriate concept in view of the ongoing co-operation between Croatia and NATO, as outlined above, as well as in view of the policies of the Alliance itself. NATO is an Alliance necessarily geared towards much more unpredictable challenges brought about by this post-cold war age. From this point of view, advancement in both security and science (and medicine) will make the world a safer place.

The Future of the Military Medical Services in NATO

Roger VAN HOOF

Major General, MD, Chairman COMEDS, Committee of the Chiefs of Military Medical Services in NATO, Secretariat: Department of Strategy, Headquarter Belgian Armed Forces, Everestreet 1, B 1140 Brussels, Belgium

This paper reflects only the view of the author
The paper was presented at the Advanced Research Workshop «Remote Cardiology Consultations Using Advanced Medical Technology – Applications for NATO Operations», held in Zagreb, Croatia 13-16 September 2005

1. Introduction

Since none of us has the perfect crystal ball, this can only be an attempt to look a few years ahead and sense what current and foreseeable developments in society, in the military and in medicine could mean for our profession as military medics.
 Which are the trends and evolutions we can see and foresee today which will inevitably become the future challenges for our younger colleagues?

To build up a strategy and strategic objectives one has inevitably to make an analysis of the future environment.

After a short review of the main characteristics in the military and in the medico military world during the Cold War - or shall we name it the Old War - I will overview briefly the changes we recently noticed in the medico military world, changes that on the one hand are caused to a great extent by external and internal transformation factors in NATO and on the other hand by fast evolving technical changes in the civilian medical world.

Finally, I will then discuss the possible role telemedicine, telecardiology and other advanced technologies can play in the future military medical operational support.

2. NATO in the (C)old War Era: 'Static' Armed Forces

NATO has spent decades in the so-called "Cold War Era". This period was characterised by the mutual nuclear deterrent and a vast geographical spread of numerous army divisions along a static border. The enemy was "doctrinally foreseeable" and Alliances were fixed.

Nations, and especially the European nations, supported this situation; they considered it as part of their home defence. They provided the necessary budgets to fully equip their armed forces. Manpower was not a problem while draft systems were in place. Operational plans anticipated huge casualty rates in case of a major combat between these heavily armed and mechanised forces. However, the mutual nuclear deterrent, a predictable way to mutually assured destruction, worked.

3. Medical Support During the Cold War Era

In most of the NATO countries, medical support of the numerous army divisions had to be organised in a known operational theatre, with known health risks and known supply and evacuation routes, using pre-known scenarios.

Medical support had to be build up gradually using also reserves and consisting of: numerous medical companies, field hospitals (mobile, semi mobile, forward, backward).

Nations had series of field hospitals under tents which needed massive reserves call up and were to support static defence lines. The draft system and the reserve troops allowed the presence of nearly all kinds of medical specialties within these field hospitals. There was no need to seek advice at home, nearly every advice was locally available.

Until little more than a decade ago, military medical support, from role 1 to role 4, was a pure national responsibility and focussed basically on Article 5 mass casualty planning. Multinational medical assets were not in the phrasebook of the average staff officer and medic in these days.

The military medical support was primarily a logistics driven requirement, emphasizing more on quantities than on technical quality.

One of the results is that in most nations, medical was considered as a sub function of logistics which main task was described as "maintaining manpower ".

Outside the operational theatre, at home, military medical support was organised in various ways in the different countries, depending on the type of national health security system.

In some countries, military medical facilities were open to the civilians, and this generated substantial financial income. In other countries the military medical service only treated military people and all costs were to be provided by the Ministry of Defence.

4. The Medical Profession During the Cold War

During the sixties and the seventies, medicine was not so expensive as it is today. Only limited medical techniques were used. Cardiac coronarography for example only started in the early seventies.

There were general practitioners, surgeons and a few anaesthesiologists, specialist in internal medicine, gynaecologists, paediatricians and a few other smaller specialties. Most of them had only a limited number of technical procedures available.

Subspecialties, such as gastro-enterologists or cardiac surgeons, for example, were only found in quite a few academic hospitals.

Military medical services financially could afford such basic medical structures, with all possible specialists and with such limited medical activities at all levels.

5. And Then Came 'the Transformation' of NATO

Since the collapse of the former WARSAW Pact, which culminated in the fall of the BERLIN Wall and the whole Iron Curtain, the economical, social, political, strategic and health environment has profoundly changed.

Over hardly a decade, the speed of change within our societies has increased dramatically.

Some of the most striking phenomena affect fundamentally, both as individuals and as societies, our perception of the hazards that may hamper our safety, well-being and way of life.

6. Change of Economical Environment

After the fall of the Berlin Wall, a lot of NATO Armed Forces were faced with three major challenges: falling defence budgets, or frozen defence budgets in a economic recession period; rising costs of both equipment and personnel, especially when the draft systems was turned into professional armed forces and demands or more spending caused by the increasing new roles and missions in NATO.

After the end of the cold war a lot of NATO nations perceived no longer the direct threats to their national security.

Nations were eager to collect the so called 'peace dividend".

A lot of nations get rid of their draft system and lowered or, in the best cases, freezed their defence budgets.

However, the transition in most nations to an all-volunteer force has driven the manpower cost but also the cost for new specialised material, especially while in a professional army there is more involvement of specialists and experts.

Most armed forces have a massive shopping list for both new equipment and personnel, which far exceeds the available financial means. As a result, not all the requirements can be met and harsh choices are to be made. One of the items on that list are requirements for advanced technologies such as network enabling capacities, part of this being Telemedicine.

But, unfortunately, most of the time the military medical services don't appear at the top of the priority shopping list, although in PSO, humanitarian aid and CIMIC activities organized by the Combat Service Support units become more and more important.

For equipment, the choice might be cancellation or delay of new programmes or smaller orders.

With a frozen or a shrinking budget, an all-volunteer force causes a shift of the ideal distribution of the budget expenditure between personnel, functioning and investments towards personnel to the detriment of necessary investments.

So, there were rising costs but there were also demands for additional money. The first impression after the fall of the Berlin Wall was that the national and international security was more guaranteed and that there was more peace in the world than ever before.

However, after a couple of years, NATO found her armed forces involved in more international crises than before and as a consequence, there were also demands for more money.

7. Change of Social Environment

The more frequent military operations abroad were caused by one concomitant social factor which changed profoundly the politico-military environment.
It was the unprecedented globalisation and interdependence of human activity.

This leads to increased mutual contacts and mobility of people, goods and ideas so that lingering crises somewhere in the world indirectly can affect supply lines of energy, stock markets, weather patterns, global economy and finally jobs in other parts of the world. The increased mutual contacts and mobility can even directly confront people with terrorism, in their own country or sometimes abroad, in their daily life for example when taking their next business or holiday flight.

Added to that is the incredible expansion of web accessible information and E mail contacts.

Today hundreds of millions of almost instantaneous individual information exchanges take place, without any state authority controlling this.

This is an incredible factor of freedom, but unfortunately also an enormous risk factor.

For the quality of the information can be quite poor and the mass magnitude of this medium can turn it into a real psycho shock wave, which is an identified prime terrorist goal.

Let alone the so called "cyber attacks", that can virtually paralyse entire sectors of society. Defending against these hazards has become a multi billion business.

Add to this the fact that there is a diagnosed "democratic deficit" in an increasing number of inter- and multinational organizations. This phenomenon is exacerbated by the lack of accountability for decisions taken by multinationals and by the global networking of organised crime.

All these factors lead to a de facto decreasing influence by the individual states on the course of action in crucial domains, such as defence, finance, and even provision of welfare.

At the same time, this situation increases the likelihood that relatively small states, or non-states actors, organizations or groups of extremist use asymmetric means, in order to impose their political or financial aims on a global scale and emphasize the need for internationalization of the defence actions.

While conventional war will remain the mean of last resort to resolve inter-state confrontations, the majority of future conflicts will be asymmetrical. Even without further proliferation, some states are known to have WMD today.

Moreover, sociologists predict increasing international competition for shrinking natural resources, such as water and energy, and they fear this will boost instability in major parts of the globe.

The rise of non-state threats is a tremendous problem for Western governments and militaries, because traditional means of deterrence fail and we are legally and behaviourally prepared to fight other legal-basis states but we are not prepared to fight terrorists.

Furthermore, the reluctance within our western type nations to cope with the inevitable casualties of conflict is a well-known weakness worldwide. This makes terrorist of guerrilla type actions causing lots of casualties the more attractive for those who are economical and militarily in the underdog situation.

In all this it obviously is crucial to "win the media war". Media coverage now has a dramatic effect on public opinion, morale of troops and finally on political sustainability within worldwide coalitions.

8. Change of Strategic and Political Environment

The period of the 'Cold War Era' was first followed by a 'hot' period of NATO led operations. They started in the early nineties in the BALKANS and they are still ongoing.

This is the Era of the Peace Support Operations with quite different characteristics.

After having agreed, or forced to agree by the multinational community to a peaceful end of a war situation a multinational force separates belligerents. They gradually evolve under military presence and political guidance towards a peaceful cohabitation.

These ongoing peace support operations continue, as a shared burden and this contrast sharply with the downsizing of the post Cold War Forces by NATO nations and with the frozen or downsized national defence budgets.

Furthermore these frequent peace supporting operations overtax military personnel and material.

The result is usually shortages in personnel and thus over-stretched, longer periods away from home and a greater willingness to substitute active duty personnel by reserves and civilians or even new advanced technologies, or to outsource some of the military activities to civil companies.

9. Transformation of NATO: Internal Factors

Confronted to all these external factors, NATO members started the internal transformation. *Transformation of NATO itself:*The NATO summit in PRAGUE set out the new beacons for the trans-Atlantic alliance in the new security environment.

It stated: "NATO needs the capability to field forces that can move quickly to wherever they are needed and sustain operations over great distance, including in an environment where they might be faced with biological, chemical and nuclear weapons."

This declaration ended the 'out of area' debate in NATO.

NATO is now involved in its first out of area operation in AFGHANISTAN.

NATO launched several initiatives: first the Defence Capability Initiatives and later on the Prague Capability Commitments.

A key evolution within this new approach now is the creation of the NATO Response Force, which is designed to operate in a high intensity environment. It will be kept at short notice, will be sustainable on its own for at least 30 days and will be able to draw on designated specialist capabilities, including a dedicated CBNR battalion. Multinational units are the key in the NATO Response Force and these multinational assets will have to train together and have to be accredited, before being accepted as operational.

10. Transformation of the Military in Nations

The new PSO missions forced many European Allies to create smaller, lighter, more mobile Forces, which are sustainable over longer periods.

The war in IRAQ showed us again the increasing use of remotely controlled precision weapons, and a dramatic evolution towards network-centric warfare techniques. A crisis is not won anymore by only the force of large Armed Forces.

However, the IRAQ war showed us also that despite a quick dismantling of the classical military means of the adversary, keeping the peace in regions where the population is traditionally armed, can pose a serious and costly challenge in both forces needed and casualties suffered. And casualties are the primary concern of the military medical services.

The trend to downsize the national Armed Forces and to make them smaller, lighter and more mobile makes logistics, medical and general infrastructure to pay more within shrinking defence budgets.

In operations, military authorities try to reduce the 'logistics footprint'. This pushes the combat service support functions to adopt ever 'lighter' and more flexible solutions. Such as the implementation of the civilian "just in time delivery" principle on military logistics and the options for outsourcing (example: third party logistics support) and off the shelf commercial solutions.

So the 'lean and mean' force, focussed mainly on the combatant core business of the future is coming up quickly.

11. Change of Health Environment

Important factors that influenced especially the transformation of the military medical services NATO were the changes in the civilian medical world and the changes of the health environment. Since the sixties and the seventies the health environment changed profoundly, especially in the Western world.Huge progression has been achieved in the medical world. Medicine becomes more and more sophisticated, more and more technical and more and more expensive. The medical domains become more and more focussed on smaller but more detailed parts. The general surgeon, anaesthesiologist, gynaecologist, paediatrician, the global expert in internal medicine are replaced by high level specialists with a very restricted domain of expertise.The health care systems in the different countries are confronted to deeper and deeper financial debts. National health care systems undergo budgetary pressures to promote new techniques, which should produce more outpatient care and shorten hospitalisation periods. National health care systems try also to limit the high technological assets in order to lower their expenses.

Most of the military medical services have tremendous difficulties to follow this trend, embedded as they are in the military structures, confronted to budget restrictions and shortages in personnel. The military medical services try to overcome these difficulties by collaborating with or even outsourcing to the civilian medical world, especially their medical support activities in the home country.

Management of the medical structures, and thus also of the military medical structures becomes more and more complicated.

In the past the commander of military medical structures at home was nearly always a physician, the complexity of the actual remaining military medical structures at home forces the military authorities to give the lead of these structures to real managers, leaving the physicians and other medical personnel more and more as medical technicians and medical advisers.

In an environment with shrinking possibilities for medical technical experience, these medical technicians are now pushed to work part time in civilian structures in order to retain their experiences.

Use of advanced technology is also evolving in medicine and health matters. Telemedicine and teleconsulting techniques as well as medical data transmission continue to develop. These means offer 'off the shelf solutions' for situations where scarce medical staffs should be engaged in more cost-efficient ways. To implement all this advanced technology, military medical services have to claim and defend their part in the national military investments.

Health environment evolved also from mostly curative activities to important preventive actions.

In most nations, armed forces personnel (military and civilian) expect a health care at home and abroad, equivalent to the national civilian health care standards.

In civilian health care, ever more emphasis is put on preventive action in order to reduce morbidity as a whole.

In military health care, growing sensitivities of the troops and the public opinion for the long-term health hazards of the operational environment are the reasons why we observe an increasing need for medical preventive actions, before, during and after deployment.

A positive evolution is a better understanding within the military of the importance to take care of pre- and post-deployment health issues. Preventive measures and reconnaissance and post deployment screening can substantially reduce both the occurrence and consequences of deployment related health issues. Medical planning activities, such as prior evaluation of the medical treatment possibilities of the Host Nation, the possibilities and constraints of medical evacuation means in the unknown operational theatre, the environmental health threats, and so on, are becoming very important.

In the operational theatre this complexity drives the military medical services further and further away from the pure logistic activities, even if in some countries medical still remains a part of logistics.

12. Transformation of the Medical Services

The same factors that influence the transformation of NATO are to be taken into account in the transformation of the medical services: falling defence budgets, rising costs, smaller, lighter, more mobile forces making more frequent tours of duty, reduction of logistics footprint

So the inevitable trend to do more with less is likely to influence the medical units too.

On the one hand military medical services are forced by the military authorities to reduce their assets.

Facing shrinking defence budgets and manpower ceilings, many NATO nations tend to progressively transfer manpower from combat service support functions, including medical, to combat and combat support functions.

We also see that military decision makers, quite naturally tend to minimise health and medical support matters, especially in the planning phase of operations.

Nations' last decades Crises Response Operation (CRO) experiences, fortunately, confirm the impression that CRO casualty rates are strikingly low, although local mass casualty situations can never be excluded.

Indeed, disease and non-operational injuries (like traffic accidents) formed the bulk of the operational medical workload in the Balkans. Lessons learned from Afghanistan and Iraq will certainly correct this picture, although, disease and non-operational injuries have been the biggest killers during any war or crisis.

Taking into account that casualties mean some degree of defeat or failure and medical support installations are a considerable logistic burden to move and support, operational planners generally tend to see things too optimistically.

The recent history told us that, due to these factors - shrinking defence budgets, absence of mass casualties and minimizing health support matters - nations were happy to silently collect the peace dividend and... medical paid twice: once as normal part of the overall force reduction, a second time since a pure restrictive interpretation of the medical tasks in CRO learned that the "small footprint" for medical was quite acceptable without consequences.

But how can this be in concordance with the fact that changes of strategic, social and health environment put to day more challenges and demands on the medical operational support and that at the same time, the political leadership, public opinion, the operational commander and the individual soldier and his family expect nothing less than the top performance to reduce the number and the consequences of casualties, applying the same quality of care as in their homeland?

As you all know, peacetime standards of timely evacuation and adequate treatment of the individual casualty, govern the number and the location of medical installations deployed, the medical people and the evacuation means needed. But not only during deployment, also for pre-, per- and post-deployment health assessments, a substantial number of medical people and important means, such as predeployment reconnaissance, epidemiologic analysing techniques, electronic communication means, and so on, are needed but are in most cases not taken into account during the operational planning.

The result is a mostly thin medical operational support, with overstressed medical people.

Thus the scarce, highly qualified and difficult to recruit medical personnel is facing more and more frequent operational tours of duty, interfering with their normal high workload in peacetime hospitals.

In most cases they must experience the frustrating situation of technical underemployment during their deployment tours, unless they have the chance to be involved in local humanitarian actions.

Severe recruitment problems and premature medical staff departures indicate today that the operational rotation frequencies of remaining scarce active duty staffs are now beyond acceptable limits in peacetime.

Medical support concepts will have to focus ever more on supporting smaller, more mobile units, equipped with greater precision firepower. This might imply the need to push forward life saving techniques to smaller units levels, especially in Special Forces type operations. This evolution pushes medical support further on the road of early stabilising techniques and consequent early medical evacuation.

Medical support installations providing the comprehensive package of all specialist care in the operational theatre will become ever more rare an asset. They will increasingly be found in modular and containerised task tailored formats on board of support ships or as host nation support facilities in adjacent countries or they will be partly or totally replaced by technology such as telemedicine, telesurgery, and so on.

All these factors: shortage of personnel, shortage of budget and material force NATO and nations to organise multinational integrated medical units (MIMU), to think about outsourcing and to apply advanced technologies.

The scarceness of medical personnel has now become the driving factor to speed up the multinational integration of medical support structures but also the use of advanced technologies such as telemedicine, teleconsulting, telesurgery.

The more complex, the more technical, the more expensive health care becomes, the more difficult it will be for military medical services to cover the whole range of military medical support in the operational theatre even in multinational assets.

Telemedicine and teleconsulting could overcome this problem and can even be organized on a multinational base also to support the smaller size, even level one, medical support units.

We should, however be aware of the trap.

Greater efficiency due to multinational cooperation is a positive evolution, but should not become the national excuse to further erode national medical capabilities into real operational showstoppers.

The need for operational medical support has to be balanced against the need for medical support in the home country. Of course, the more complex, the more technical, the more expensive health care is, the more difficult it becomes for military medical services to cover the whole range of medical support at home. So cooperation with and even outsourcing to the civilian sector seems logic. But these decisions should always be guided by the need for experienced medical personnel in the operational theatre.

Finally: what are the future challenges for the implementation of Telemedicine in the military medical structures? I will briefly mention the challenges in three domains:

- Budget
- Communications system
- Standardization

Budget: Military medical authorities should also be aware of the fact that removing high qualified medical personnel from the operational list is much easier to do than to persuade the military authorities to allocate a substantial part of the investments for overall military advanced technology to the military medical domain.

Communications system: Telemedicine and teleconsulting mean not only the acquisition of expensive material but also need the guarantee that part of the military operational telecommunication systems can be used by the medical service. In many cases, military authorities don't understand this.

As you probably all know, the use by medical units of real time telecommunications for telemedicine purposes during the military operational activities may be a big problem. Military authorities are not so prepared to allow the use of 'their' operational telecommunication systems by the medics. And a distinct 'medical telecommunication system' is in most cases not available due to budget restrictions.

And we only speak here about telemedicine and teleconsulting. But what if, in the future, these evolve to technologies such as real time telesurgery? Will the medical services be able to get the money and the necessary telecommunication systems for this in the future?

Standardization: Especially while telemedicine and teleconsulting techniques can be used in a multinational environment, standardization is a prerequisite. In recent years a lot of initiatives have been taken by different NATO panels and workgroups to try to standardize the Telemedicine process. It started with the Telemedicine panel established by the General Medical Working Group under the Joint Standardisation Board of NATO. This panel collaborates now with the Medical Information Management Systems working group of COMEDS, now renamed as MedCis working group.

Justification of Investing in Telemedicine

Spase VULIĆ[a], Nives KLAPAN[b]

[a]*Program Director, The Ministry of Health and Social Welfare - Health System Project, Zagreb, Croatia*
[b]*Department of Telemedicine, Zagreb, Croatia*

The paper was presented at the Advanced Research Workshop «Remote Cardiology Consultations Using Advanced Medical Technology – Applications for NATO Operations», held in Zagreb, Croatia 13-16 September 2005

1. Summary

Justification of investing in Telemedicine can be perceived through two presentations of case-studies.

The first case-study deals with the use of Telemedicine in Radiology. The network connecting county Departments for Radiology with reference centres at the Neuro-surgical clinics indicates that 40% of all consulted patients can be treated at county hospitals, thus resulting in savings on travel expenses etc.

The other study is also based on savings resulting from the use of Telemedicine, concerning travel expenses and daily allowances as well as evasion of repeated consultations and charges.

The aforementioned studies prove that Telemedicine is economically cost-efficient and medically successful.

Implementation of telemedicine worldwide and in Croatia is a result of breakthrough of sophisticated medical technology, communications and IT support.

A completely new meaning and contents is given to the new technology that is used in TLM (*telemedicine*), because when supported by the other technological solutions that technology is providing service on distance by transferring images, sounds and other signals. The expensive technology that has been causing the increases of medical expenses so far, nowadays thanks to its new role, or so called "positive paradox", is decreasing expenses in diagnostics and treatments and is increasing the efficiency of medical service.

Table 1: Number of referrals in polyclinic institutions 1996 – 2003 (irregular distribution of patients)

	Year of referral	Number of referrals in polyclinic	Index 1996 = 100
1	1996	5.277.237	100
2	1997	5.649.999	127
3	2000	6.598.913	125
4	2001	6.757.771	128
5	2002	7.003.784	133
6	2003	7.038.521	135

Source: Croatian national institute of public health, Croatian health services 1996 – 2003

The number of referrals in polyclinic health care shows a tendency of a constant growth and has almost a linear growth trend from 1996 to 2002, what can be seen in the Table 1. The growth index of referrals in the year 2002 is 133 which, in comparison with the ones in 1996, proves that the transfer of patients from PHC (*Primary health care*) in a five-year period has grown for a third. This phenomenon is rather disturbing since the growth of population failed to show the same dynamics - the number of inhabitants stagnates or has improved slightly due to a number of come backs, but this is not perceived as being significant enough for the analysis.

2. Where is the Solution?

The solution is in radically reorganizing health care system and in introducing telemedicine. The implementation of new technology in health service system is a requirement of time we live in because only the telemedicine combined with new technology can contribute to real reform of the health system.The first results of TLM usage in radiology are encouraging (Table 2).
It has been documented that out of total number of 100 provided consultations in average 40 % of the total does not require any further treatment or medical service, which results with high savings in travel expenses, daily allowances, etc.
If the distance is bigger the implementation of TLM is more profitable.

Table 2: Savings on transport costs by use and non-use of telemedicine in year 2000 in the field of Radiology

No. of hospitals	No. of referrals in TLM	Number of patients that		% of patients in column 4	Distance from hospital to RFC Zagreb x 2	Savings	
		Use RFC	Do not use RFC			col. 4 x col. 6 in km	col. 7 x 28,00
1	2	3	4	5	6	7	8
14	752	427	315	41,89	312	98,244	2.750.832

Summary version; Source: Reference centre for telemedicine, annual report for 2002

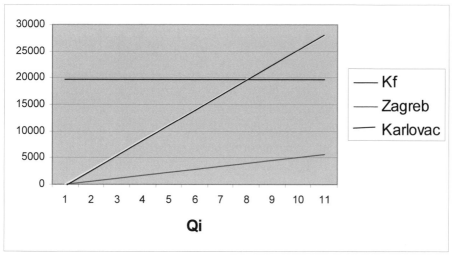

Figure 1: The threshold for investing in Zagreb and Karlovac

In 1998, the total of 33 sets of telemedical equipment, transmitting CT scans into the main reference centre of the Neurology clinic in Zagreb, were installed in 18 counties throughout Croatia. The results of 15 workstations show that:

Out of the total of 752 consultations, 437 patients or 58,11% were referred to a higher level, whereas 41,89% remained on the level of primary health care. Considering the transport costs, this meant saving of 2.750.832 kn or 423.204 US$.

It is worth mentioning that a single workstation cost the total of 85.000 kn or 13.076 US$. Thus, the cost of 33 workstations amounts to:

$$85.000 \times 33 = 2.805.000 \text{ kn or } 431.538 \text{ US\$}.$$

Therefore, with only 14 workstations in operation, the entire investment would generate return in almost a year. With all 33 workstations in operation, the savings will enlarge.Based on this data, the threshold for investing in telemedicine has been calculated. The charts show that in telemedicine the distance has a positive effect on the decrease of expenses.

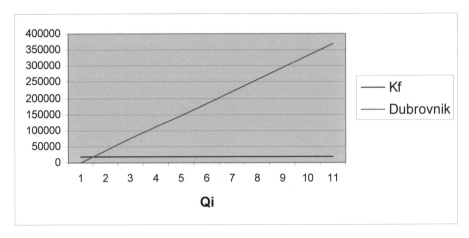

Figure 2: The threshold for investing in Dubrovnik

In Zagreb, at least 9 patients are needed to reach the threshold for investing in telemedicine, whereas in Dubrovnik, due to great distances and saving on transport expenses, the threshold for investing in telemedicine is 1,5 patients (based on Table 2).
A few words about application of telemedicine on islands and benefits that can be expected.The strategy of health system development which is currently under way will stress the problems of medicine on islands. Therefore, the strategy of health reform on Croatian islands should be based on upgrading the efficiency of health system through redefining the priorities, along with improved availability and quality of health services, by planned utilization of telecommunication – telemedicine, that should be implemented according to modern telecare in this country.

Many benefits are expected from application of telemedicine at islands, such as:

- sparing patients from travel, wasting time and absenteeism, along with upgraded medical care quality
- better communication between primary health care and higher levels
- assistance to G.P. in emergency and life threatening states
- sense of security for patients and inhabitants of the islands in general
- better and proper diagnoses of the patient

General medicine services at islands
- saving costs -
Result of examination (see Table 3)
Total number of examined persons in primary health care: 233.634
Referred to the higher level polyclinic: 62.603 = 27% (state average is 33%)
Total number of patients treated in PHC: 171.031
Total number of patients: 62.603 x   40%   of referrals
$$= \ 25.041 \ \text{patients}$$
25.041 + 171.031   =   196.072   patients could be treated at the PHC (82,92%)
Financially, result = savings of   1.198.115 USD
- 30 % of the costs
838.681 USD   netto

Table 3: General medicine services at islands

	ISLAND (Place)	No. of clinics	No. of insurants	No. of visits	No. of referrals	% of referrals	40% of referrals
1	2	3	4	5	6	7	8
1.1	KORČULA (Korčula)	7	6416	40378	10272	25.43	4108
1.2	(Blato)	3	2939	28176	5619	19.94	2247
1.3	(Vela Luka)	1	875	4578	2176	47.47	868
1.4	(Smokvica)	4	2862	12897	5863	45.46	235
2.1	BRAČ (Bol)	2	1576	12656	2762	21.82	1105
2.2	(Milna)	1	742	5574	700	12.55	280
2.3	(Postira)	1	1137	3634	1138	31.31	455
2.4	(Pučišća)	2	1931	14830	2068	13.94	827
2.5	(Supetar)	2	3415	21274	6292	29.58	2516
2.6	(Sutivan)	1	1602	8142	2296	28.19	918
3.1	HVAR (Hvar)	3	2752	24960	4256	17.05	1702
3.2	(Jelsa)	3	4089	14326	6638	46.34	2655
3.3	(Stari Grad)	2	2496	18458	4855	26.30	1942
3.4	(Sućuraj)	1	499	4874	1203	24.68	481
4.1	VIS (Vis)	2	1544	10052	3279	32.62	1311
4.2	(Komiža)	2	1888	8825	3186	36.10	1274
	TOTAL	**37**	**36763**	**233634**	**62603**	**27.00**	**25041**

Source: Croatian National Institute of Public Health, annual report.

Indirect savings:
Indirect savings on travel fees in average
$$150 \text{ kn} \times 25\,041 = 3.756.150 \text{ kn} \quad \text{or} \quad 577.869 \text{ USD}$$
Transportation costs which are in average cca 200 kn per person,
$$\text{saving } 5.008.200 \text{ kn} \quad \text{or} \quad 770.493 \text{ USD}$$
Total expense for unnecessary consultations amounts to 1.198.115 + 577.869 + 770.493
$$= 2.546.477 \text{ USD}$$

By using Telemedicine saving per patient is 102 USD. Therefore, we can conclude that telemedicine is economically affordable, medically effective and socially acceptable.

References

[1] A model for Evaluating the Cost Impact of Telemedicine As Compared to Face – to – Face, title://A:/AMODEL-1.HTM, October 31, 2002

[2] Bartolić, A., Jonjić, A. Social Medicine, Handbook of seminar exercises, 4th edition, Medical Faculty Rijeka, Rijeka, October 1994

[3] Bartolić, A. Health Care in the Pazin area, Pazin, 2003

[4] Benc, S. Metodological suitability and practical use of Cost-benefit analysis in Croatian Economy, doctoral dissertation, Zagreb, December 1997

[5] Financing of health services, Report of a WHO Study Group, Technical Report Series, 625, World Health Organization, Geneva, 1978

[6] Annual report on Health Insurance and Health Care of the Republic of Croatia in 2001 – Financial plan and underlying assumptions of business for 2002, Croatian Institute for Health Insurance, April 2002

[7] Health 21 – health for all in the 21st century, an Introduction, European Health for All Series No 5, World Health Organization, Regional Office for Europe, Copenhagen, 1998

[8] Health Economics – A Programme for Action, Division of Strengthening of Health Services, World Health Organization, Geneva, 1988

[9] Annual report for 2000, Croatian National Institute of Public Health, Zagreb, 2001

[10] Annual report for 2001, Croatian National Institute of Public Health, Zagreb, 2002

[11] Annual report for 2002, Croatian National Institute of Public Health, Zagreb, 2003

[12] Journal of Telemedicine and Telecare, TeleMed 2001, Eight International Conference on Telemedicine and Telecare, London, 15 – 16 January 2001, Telemedicine Forum of the Royal Society of Medicine Press LTD, London, 2001

[13] Paladino, J. Application of Telemedicine in Referral Centre for Neuro-surgery, Medicinar, Students' journal of the Medical Faculty in Zagreb, Vol. 41., No. 1, Medicine edition, Zagreb, December 1999, 74

[14] Radiology and Imaging, Hospital Healthcare Europe 2001/2002, CAMPDEN publishing LTD, London, 2002

[15] Sharma, S. Economics does Matter: About Economics and Economists (Selected works), Mikorad – Zagreb, 2002

[16] Skupnjak, B., Vulić, S. Some International Experiences and Recommendations related to reforms in the Health Care System, doc. mat., Med-Ekon, Zagreb, 2003

[17] Skupnjak, B., Vulić, S., Šimunec, D., Božan Mihelčić, V. The Development of Nursing in the Context of New Regulations, Nurse journal, No. 3, Zagreb, 2003, 13-18

[18] Telemedicine in Croatia, editors-in-chief: Klapan, I., Čikeš, I., Medika, Zagreb, 2001

[19] Vulić, S. Health in Transition, Observatory London

[20] Vuletić, S. Teleradiology network of CT and MR equipment in Croatian hospitals, paper for master's degree, University of Zagreb, 2001

Telecardiology - Patterns for Current and Future Use

Ståle WALDERHAUG[a,b], Per Håkon MELAND[a]

[a] *Research Scientist, Norwegian Joint Medical Service, MEDOPS/Ulleväl University Hospital, OSLO MIL/Akershus, 0015 Oslo, Norway*
[b] *Research Scientist, SINTEF ICT, SP Andersensvei 15b, 7465 Trondheim, Norway*

The paper was presented at the Advanced Research Workshop «Remote Cardiology Consultations Using Advanced Medical Technology – Applications for NATO Operations», held in Zagreb, Croatia 13-16 September 2005

Abstract. Telecardiology is a telemedicine service that can provide expert consultation and life-supporting treatment to patients independent of geographical location. The required technology has been available for many years, but the diffusion of telecardiology services is still limited. With the aging population of the industrial world and the increase of chronically ill patients, there is a need for telecardiology services. This paper presents a survey on how telecardiology services are being used today. The survey was conducted by reviewing articles published in recognized journals and conferences and categorizing them according to a telemedicine taxonomy, which was extended for telecardiology purposes. Based on the survey results, interoperability issues are discussed and also how standardization may change the pattern for use of telecardiology. Our principal results are that very few publications describe mobile telecardiology services that facilitate wireless communication. More research needs to be conducted on mobile telecardiology services and interoperability issues on information and communication levels must be worked out.

1. Introduction

Telecardiology [1]services have been provided since the early 1900 when experiments using telephone were described in The diffusion of telecardiology services is limited taken into account the amount of research and development that has been carried out since the first telecardiology services were introduced[2]. With an aging population and an increase in cardiovascular diseases, the need for telecardiology services will increase; according to Frost and Sullivan there will be over 4 million cardiac patients in Europe being remotely monitored by 2011 [3]. This will require a considerable diffusion of high quality telecardiology services.

Technical barriers influence the implementation and deployment of operational telecardiology services. Telecardiology services necessitate information sharing between two or more actors. Information is captured by a local user with a medical device and sent to a remote user for review and analysis. If the local user has no information about the hardware and software components the remote user applies, standardization and *interoperability* is a requisite for correct operation. To overcome these potential problems and provide *interoperable* services, standardization and extensive research is needed. Tanriverdi and Iacono discuss the barriers to diffusion of telemedicine services in [4]. Here they argue that the reason for the low diffusion is a combination of technical, economic, organizational and behavioral barriers. A large portion of the technical barriers that limit the diffusion of telemedicine are related to transmission of information between system hardware and software components. An ECG device hooked up to a wired or wireless communication line should send what you see locally to the remote site in a way that enables remote user share your view. Unfortunately this is not always the case because of lack of standardization or that existing standards are unclear[5].

Current research on information systems, communication technology and computer supported collaborative work in medicine will affect the structure of telecardiology services in the next decades. In what way it will affect the structure is not easy to predict. In our background research we have not found any scientific publications that have investigated the global status of telecardiology services research with respect to application purpose, service configuration and information technology applied. This information is a prerequisite for discussing the future telecardiology services, thus there is a need to conduct a survey on what research have been and are being done in the area of telecardiology. The survey can be used to identify areas where more research is needed in order to promote more and better telecardiology services.

We use scientific literature search engines to identify scientific work published in the most recognized journals and conferences. By reviewing this scientific work we address the following questions:

- What are the current patterns for use of telecardiology services?
- How do interoperability issues affect these patterns?
- What will be future patterns for use of telecardiology services?

Our main result is that telecardiology is mainly used in static configurations such as hospital to hospital consultations. Based on current status of telecardiology services, new technological development and the need for interoperable services, we conclude that future use of telecardiology services will be more mobile and dynamically configurable. The paper will first present the method for our research. Then we present the results and classification before we discuss the outcome with respect to interoperability and future use of telecardiology. We do not evaluate the services' outcome as this has been done in previous publications such as [6-14].

2. Materials and Methods

2.1. Search and Selection

A methodical literature survey in the field of telecardiology has been conducted. This was done by using some of the major electronic literature index databases, namely Google Scholar[1], IngentaConnect[2],

---

[1] Google Scholar: http://scholar.google.com/

[2] IngentaConnect: http://www.ingentaconnect.com/

PubMed/MEDLINE[3], ACM Portal Digital Library[4], ISI Web of Science[5] and IEEE Xplore[6]. These are considered to be the main search engines for scientific publications in medical and computer science research. The goal was to establish a representative selection of scientific articles in the area of telecardiology, not to review everything that has ever been published. This allowed us to only include articles written in the English and those available in an electronic format. The search terms were "telecardiology", "telemedicine AND cardiology", "remote cardiology", "tele-electrocardiography", "tele-ECG", "tele-echocardiography" and variations of these. We chose only to include articles where telecardiology was the main topic, not general telemedicine articles where telecardiology was one (of many) application area(s). Articles from both medical and computer science journals/conferences were considered.

The index databases returned about 450 results. Because of a large amount of overlap between them, it is difficult to give an exact number. The initial screening of these articles was based on title, abstract and keywords. All abstracts were read and classified by both authors, and when this information was not sufficient for classification, full-text versions were obtained for a closer inspection. Discrepancies between the authors were discussed until agreement. References to some other central articles that were not found in the initial search were also examined and included. Obvious article duplications were excluded. A total of 94 articles and reports were identified as relevant and reviewed.

2.2. Classification

The selected articles were classified according to a telemedicine taxonomy published by Tulu[15], which we extended and specialized for telecardiology. The taxonomy is a useful method to compare and contrast different studies end efforts in the field of telecardiology. From Tulu's taxonomy we included *clinical and non-clinical application purpose, environmental settings, telecommunication technologies and bandwidth* and *delivery options*. These parameters enabled us to answer "why", "where" and "how". All parameters had zero or more entries for each article.

We chose to add some more details to the taxonomy to be able to distinguish between computer science and medical research ("what") and to see geographical distribution and evolution of articles over time ("when"). Since telecardiology includes many types of *clinical information* that are associated with very different communication infrastructure, we added a parameter for this based on the categories of capturing devices defined in by Telemedical.com Inc[7] (one study may include more than one information type). All the selected articles were registered and the classifications coded into a database. If some of these parameters were not described in the article, this was registered as blank. The final taxonomy used for our classification is listed in appendix A.

---

[3] PubMed: http://www.ncbi.nlm.nih.gov/entrez/

[4] The ACM Digital Library: http://portal.acm.org/

[5] ISI Web of Science: http://www.isinet.com/products/citation/wos/

[6] IEEE Xplore: http://ieeexplore.ieee.org/Xplore/

[7] Telemedical.com Inc: http://telecardiology.info/

2.3. Data analysis

The collected data was exported from the database into a spreadsheet for basic statistically analysis and comparison. This typically included combining the classification results with year published and place of origin to look for patterns and trends. Expected and obvious results are ignored further in this paper.

3. Results

Our search resulted in 94 articles that met our defined criteria. The earliest article was from 1988, but the majority of articles were published between 1999 and 2004 (11, 9, 15, 15, 13 and 12 articles respectively). Only 4 articles from 2005 were identified (but the survey was conducted during August 2005). 22 of the selected articles were from the USA, while 15 were from Italy and 9 from the UK. Australia had 6 articles while Spain, India and Greece each had 5 of the selected articles.

Of the 94 selected articles were 62 published in journals, 29 at scientific conferences and 3 articles were published elsewhere. The most represented journals were International Journal of Telemedicine and Telecare[8], Telemedicine Journal and E-health[9] and IEEE Transactions on Information Technology in Biomedicine[10]. Articles from the Computers in Cardiology[11] conference were the most frequent conference articles in our selection.

3.1. Classification according to telemedicine taxonomy

This section presents the results according to the telemedicine taxonomy. Results from the parameters *non-clinical purpose* and *delivery option* are not presented here as they have no relation to the questions being addressed in the paper.

3.2. Application purpose

From a clinical perspective, *diagnostic* and *consultation* are the two main categories (37 and 35 of the articles). *Monitoring* and *provision of specialty care* have 25 and 20 respectively. *Triage* and *supervision of specialty care* are minor applications (2 and 5 articles). None of the selected articles reported *surgical* or *non-surgical treatment* as a purpose for applying telecardiology services.

---

[8] Royal Society of Medicine Press, International Journal of Telemedicine and Telecare:
http://www.roysocmed.ac.uk/pub/jtt.htm

[9] Mary Ann Liebert Inc, Telemedicine Journal and e-Health:
http://www.liebertpub.com/publication.aspx?pub_id=54

[10] IEEE Transactions on Information Technology in Biomedicine:
http://www.vtt.fi/tte/samba/projects/titb/index.html

[11] Computers in Cardiology: http://www.cinc.org/

3.3. Environmental Settings

All the articles had *small/large hospital* (where the expert is located) as receiving environment.

With respect to sending environment (from), many articles did not make a distinction between large and small hospitals. Neither did they distinguish between outreach clinic and health center. We choose to merge these into 2 categories, namely hospital and health center. An article may report zero, one or more environmental setting, for instance both from home and small hospital. This leaves us with the following results: 21 articles sent information from a hospital. 27 of the articles sent information from a health center. 24 of the articles reported that they sent information from the patients' home while 1 article sent data from an ambulance vehicle. 13 articles described communication in a test laboratory setting and 8 articles did not give details where they sent information from (blank). None of the selected articles reported to have sent information from sea, air or field medical treatment facilities.

3.4. Communication Infrastructure

The majority of the articles based their telecardiology on *wired communication* infrastructure. Many systems could use more than one type of communication technology such as wired DSL, cable modem and high speed networks. If we look at the type of communication infrastructure applied in the period from 1988 to 2005 we will see that the use of wireless communication increases from 1999 to 2004 (2005).

With respect to wireless communication, USA has only 4% use of wireless communication while UK, Spain and Italy are using wireless communication technologies to a larger extent (57%, 45% and 27% respectively). Greece and Australia are however at the same level as USA.

3.5. Type of scientific results and special aspects for telecardiology

Cardiology involves many types of clinical information. We extended the taxonomy to capture this. If we use clinical information and origin of study we find that there is a difference between countries and continents. Looking at the top five publishing countries we find that in USA 58% of the articles included echocardiography and 15% included EKG and Holter Monitoring Devices. Echocardiography is included in 11% in Italian articles and none from the UK. EKG is included in 63% and 100% respectively. The clinical information used in telecardiology services in Spanish and Greek articles is comparable what is reported in Italian articles. Australian articles reported about 20% of both echocardiography and EKG and Holter Monitoring Devices.

4. Discussion

We have performed a methodological search for scientific telecardiology articles. We identified 94 articles that were published between 1988 and 2005. Our selection of search engines was based on popularity in the medical and computer science field. The overlap of the search results indicates that we have found the majority of scientific articles available online in English language.

4.1. Pattern for current use of telecardiology services

Looking at the application purpose we find that telecardiology is mostly used for *diagnostic, consultation, monitoring* and *provision of specialty care.* Very few articles used telecardiology for (patient or professional medical) educational purposes. Tele-teaching and tele-guiding [16] is not widely used for telecardiology, but there may be an implicit learning aspect of "provision of speciality care" even though few articles have stated this.

We also see that the number of publications on mobile use of telecardiology is very limited. Only 1 article presents a system that send information from an ambulance. No articles present telecardiology services for use in airplanes or boat/ship. Such systems must use wireless communication, and as our results indicates, wireless communication is rarely used. The fact that telecardiology services are mostly used between two fixed locations (home/health center to hospital) implies that wired communication is the most used communication infrastructure. The implication may also be the other way; limited access to wireless communication limits the development and deployment of mobile telecardiology services. Another reason may be that these kinds of telecardiology services are most successful. Both Hailey (6) and Hersh (17) report that the strongest evidence of benefit is provided by the studies of home care applications of telecardiology.

An interesting observation is that articles from USA focus much more on echocardiography than European and Australian articles. One factor that influences this may be the selected communication infrastructure. Echocardiography typically requires more bandwidth than EKG. An aspect that influences this may be the fact that USA has only 4% use of wireless communication while UK, Spain and Italy are using wireless communication technologies to a larger extent. Greece and Australia are however at the same level as USA. We have not found any other results in our material that can be used to explain this.

4.2. Telecardiology interoperability

Many articles describe that they have developed their own software to be able to communicated information and integrate into existing hospital infrastructure. The reason for this can be incompatible or inaccessible (vendor-proprietary) hardware/software interfaces. Reading structured medical information out of a monitoring device is a complex and time-consuming task. Many device manufacturers offer their own software tailored for their hardware. The medical institutions will however import the monitored information into the patients' journals and must therefore write a software "wrapper" application. If the medical institution uses hardware from many different vendors, the cost of integrating all monitoring devices into the "information backbone" will be quite high. An unambiguous standard that describes the format and protocols for communicating with cardiology devices would ease this integration and make resources available for applied medical research. OpenECG[12] is a project that seeks to standardize communication with ECG devices, thus making interoperability between hardware and software more likely.

---

[12] OpenECG Project: http://www.openecg.net/

Standardization and development of high-level interfaces to medical devices and software will be an important task to improve the flexibility and integratability of telecardiology components. With a high-level standardized interface an organization can integrate and deploy telecardiology services more effectively than today.

4.3 Future pattern for use of telecardiology services

Based on the results from our survey, the increasing need for cardiology services, and the trends in computer and communication technology, we can say that mobile wireless systems for telecardiology need more research. Very few scientific publications have until now described telecardiology services for mobile wireless use.

As new small and mobile telecardiology devices are being distributed to shopping malls, airplanes, ships, highway medical emergency stations and so on, new services will come into being. Access to high-speed wireless communication will become a matter of course as Wi-fi[13] hotspots and 3G[14] mobile technologies are being introduced into the market. With the adoption of mobile monitoring devices it is essential that they can communicate wirelessly to the best (nearest or most skilled) cardiology expert service available. This requires interoperability between monitoring devices, communication infrastructures and health information systems.

A new dimension will be added to the current static communication structure between health centers and hospitals. With these new dimensions, new requirements will evolve to support the new telecardiology services. Interoperability on communication and information levels will be key issues for the future where the old static infrastructure breaks up and is replaced by a dynamic wireless full-featured telecardiology system that can connect to the best available expert cardiology services.

References

[1] EC-IST EC: Telemedicine Glossary, 5 ed: European Commission, 2003. (Beolchi L, ed.

[2] Sending dental X-rays using telegraph. Dental Radiography and Photography 1929; 2(16).

[3] Sullivan F: Remote Patient Monitoring : A European Perspective. Frost & Sullivan, 2003.

[4] Tanriverdi H, Iacono CS: Knowledge barriers to diffusion of telemedicine. Proceedings of the international conference on Information systems, Helsinki, Finland, 1998.

[5] Chiarugi FL, P.J. Chronaki, C.E. Tsiknakis, M. Orphanoudakis, S.C.: Developing manufacturer-independent components for ECG viewing andfor data exchange with ECG devices: can the SCP-ECG standard help? Computers in Cardiology 2001, Rotterdam, Netherlands, 09/23/2001 - 09/26/2001, 2001.

[6] Hailey David OA, Roine Risto: Published evidence on the success of telecardiology: a mixed record. Journal of Telemedicine and Telecare 2004; 10(Supplement 1): 36-38.

[7] Hersh W, Helfand M, Wallace J, et al.: Telemedicine for the Medicare Population. Evidence Report/Technology Assessment No. 24. AHRQ Publication No. 01-E012. Rockville, MD: Agency for Healthcare Research and Quality; 2001.

---

[13] IEEE 802.11 homepage: http://grouper.ieee.org/groups/802/11/

[14] 3GPP homepage: http://www.3gpp.org/

[8]   Grigsby J, Sanders J: Telemedicine: where it is and where it's going. Annals of Internal Medicine 1998; 129: 123 - 127.

[9]   Balas E, Jaffrey F, Kuperman G, et al.: Electronic communication with patients evaluation of distance medicine technology. Journal of the American Medical Association 1997; 278: 152 - 159.

[10]   Ohinmaa A, Hailey D, Roine D: The Assessment of Telemedicine: General Principles and a Systematic Review. Helsinki, Finland: Finnish Office for Health Care Technology Assessment; 1999.

[11]   Almazan C, Gallo P: Assesssing Clinical Benefit and Economic Evaluation in Telemedicine. Barcelona, Spain: Catalan Agency for Health Technology Assessment; 1999.

[12]   Currell R, Urquhart C, Wainwright P, Lewis R: Telemedicine versus face to face patient care: effects on professional practice and health care outcomes. Cochrane Database of Systematic Reviews [computer file] 2000: CD002098.

[13]   Mair F, Whitten P: Systematic review of studies of patient satisfaction with telemedicine. British Medical Journal 2000; 320: 1517 - 1520.

[14]   Whitten P, Kingsley C, Grigsby J: Results of a meta-analysis of cost-benefit research: is this a question worth asking? Journal of Telemedicine & Telecare 2000; 6: S4 - S6.

[15]   Tulu B, Chatterjee S, Laxminarayan S: A Taxonomy of Telemedicine Efforts with Respect to Applications, Infrastructure, Delivery Tools, Type of Setting and Purpose. HICSS '05: Proceedings of the Proceedings of the 38th Annual Hawaii International Conference on System Sciences (HICSS'05) - Track 6, 2005.

[16]   Spruijt HJ, Dijk WA, Visscher KJ, et al.: Teleconsulting, teleguiding and teleteaching: gigabit network. Computers in Cardiology, Rotterdam, 23-26 September, 2001.

[17]   Hersh W, Helfand M, Wallace J, et al.: Clinical outcomes resulting from telemedicine interventions: a systematic review. BMC Medical Informatics and Decision Making 2001; 1(1): 5.

Table 1: Taxonomy defined by Tulu et al [15]. Parameters in italic in have been added. A parameter named "Mobile" in Environment settings has been removed and replaces by the parameters in italic.

Application purpose		Communication Technologies	Environment settings
Clinical	**Non-clinlical**	Wired Dial-Up	Large hospital
Triage	Professional Medical Education	Wired DSL	Small hospital
Diagnostic	Patient Education	Wired Cable	Outreach clinic
Non-Surgical Treatment	Research	Modem	Health center
Surgical Treatment	Public Health	Wired High Speed	Home
Consultation	Administrative	Wireless 802.11	Air (AeroMedevac)
Monitoring		2G	Sea (Naval medical facility)
Provision of Specialty Care		2,5G	Land (Field Hospital)
Supervision of Specialty Care		3G	Ambulance (land)
		Satellite	Testlaboratory
		Low band radio	

Table 2: Delivery options. The parameters in italic have been added to the taxonomy defined by Tulu et al[15].

	Synchronous	Asynchronous
Audio	Telephone Audioconferencing	Voicemail
Video	Videoconferencing	Video/audiostreaming
Data	Instant Messaging Shared Elecronic white boards Real-time data (binary)	Paging Fax Data/binary streaming Email Web pages Store and forward Web forums

Table 3: Taxonomy extensions. Information as defined by [telecardiology.info].Type of study is defined by Shaw [18]. Science is defined by the authors.

Information	Science	Type of study
Patient Symptom and Medical History Data Capture	Medical	Procedure or technique
Electronic Stethoscopes	Mathematics/signal processing	Qualitative or descriptive model
Vital Sign Monitoring Devices	Communication	Empirical model
EKG and Holter Monitoring Devices	Software	Analytic model
Defibrillators	Hardware	Tool or notation
Chemical Monitoring	Health Informatics	Specific solution, prototype, answer, or judgment
Echocardiography	Architecture	Report
Doppler Devices	Other	
Impedence Cardiography		
Video and Still Digital Cameras		
Angiography		
Other		

Remote Cardiology Consultations Using Advanced Medical Technology
I. Klapan and R. Poropatich (Eds.)
IOS Press, 2006

Author Index